Progress Notes

Progress Notes

• • • • • • •

ONE YEAR
IN THE
FUTURE
OF
MEDICINE

• • • • • • • • • • • •

ABRAHAM M. NUSSBAUM, MD

JOHNS HOPKINS UNIVERSITY PRESS | *Baltimore*

Johns Hopkins University Press

2715 North Charles Street

Baltimore, Maryland 21218

www.press.jhu.edu

Library of Congress Cataloging-in-Publication Data

Names: Nussbaum, Abraham M., 1975– author.

Title: Progress notes : one year in the future of medicine / Abraham M.
Nussbaum, MD.

Description: Baltimore : Johns Hopkins University Press, 2024. |
Includes bibliographical references and index.

Identifiers: LCCN 2023033225 | ISBN 9781421448947 (hardcover ; alk. paper) |
ISBN 9781421448954 (ebook)

Subjects: MESH: Education, Medical—methods | Curriculum |
Patient-Centered Care—methods | Students, Medical—psychology |
Physician-Patient Relations

Classification: LCC R737 | NLM W 18 | DDC 610.71/1—dc23/eng/20240102

LC record available at https://lccn.loc.gov/2023033225

A catalog record for this book is available from the British Library.

Special discounts are available for bulk purchases of this book.
For more information, please contact Special Sales at specialsales@jh.edu.

• • • • • • • • • • •

TO THE STUDENTS WHO

PROVED THEMSELVES:

CATHERINE,

ITZAM,

MACKENZIE,

MAGGIE,

MALLORY,

MEGAN,

SARAH

• • • • • • •

AND THE STUDENTS WHO

PROVED ME:

EAMON,

MARY CLARE,

AND HELENA FRANCES

• • •

*A person is never known
till a person is proved.*

—Charles Dickens, *Bleak House*

Contents

SEE ONE

*M*OST JOBS ARE JOBS. Workers trade time for money. Becoming a doctor isn't like that. Medical training can mean more time for more money, sure. But what really makes medicine different is that when you train as a doctor, you trade both time and money to be transformed into a different kind of person. The kind of person who can reach into a wound and staunch the bleeding at its root. The kind of person who can touch a surface rash and recognize it as a sign of an unseen illness inside. The kind of person who can accompany someone into or out of this life. Becoming a doctor changes how a person relates to other people. If a doctor is transformed the right way, the sick are made better by the doctor's transformation. If a doctor is transformed the wrong way, physicians and patients alike suffer.

For more than a century, the transformation for physicians like me has been about knowing the body, not the person, of the people we meet as patients. We went to the right colleges and earned the right grades in chemistry and physics to earn admittance to the best medical school that would have us. When we relocated for med school, we were taught to take apart the body's seventy-some organs, its two hundred bones, and its six hundred muscles. Our education was a textbook-of-the-body approach. Know the parts of the body, how they break, and how to reassemble them. The approach can work when you have an acute illness or injury in one of the parts that a physician, trained in one of our dozens of specialties and subspecialties, knows how to fix, but it falters when you need a physician who knows who you are and how you fit into your community.

Medical training is expensive, costing hundreds of thousands of dollars—I paid off my own student loans the summer our son went off to college. It's time-consuming—medical training lasts a minimum of seven years after college and usually takes over your twenties and sometimes your thirties as well. It's hierarchical—medicine is almost as regimented as the military, and your place is indicated by your rank. It's also outmoded—despite decades of calls for change, physicians too often follow a hoary adage: *See one, do one, teach one.* See someone else perform a procedure you haven't seen before, do the procedure yourself the next time, and then teach the procedure to the next physician. You form a chain of knowledge to which each physician adds a link.

But what of the people upon whom these procedures are seen, done, and demonstrated?

See it, do it, teach it. The logic undergirding the adage puts procedures over persons, and the logic is first imprinted when the student ritually strips personhood from a dead body. Doctors build up medical knowledge from the bodies of the dead. You see your first corpse in a cadaver lab as a first-year medical student. You look at the blank expanse of its back instead of gazing on the expressive face. You cut down, naming as you go each layer of skin (*epidermis, dermis, hypodermis*) and muscle (*trapezius, rhomboid major, serratus posterior*) instead of the labor, loss, and love it carried. Your instructor shows you how to take the body apart so that you can read its muscles, organs, and vessels for signs of disease.

While picking apart a body in the cadaver lab, I wiped formaldehyde fluids on my white polyester lab coat and listened to MP3 blogs like *Said the Gramophone*. Given how little medical school curricula have truly changed over the past century, I could have been listening to actual gramophones.

As for the hundreds of thousands of physicians before me, I picked apart a cadaver as a first-year student until it resembled the atlas of anatomy next to the dissecting table. That took months. There was the corpse whose autopsy I witnessed as a second-year student. That took an hour. And there were living patients I met as a third-year student. That took minutes, but by that point I had trouble seeing them as people rather than as bodies.

As a third-year student on trauma surgery, I bicycled in before dawn to prepare the team's patient list. I would harvest lab results, take vital signs, record the meds taken (and refused), and summarize it all in bullet points printed in seven-point font on a single piece of double-sided paper that added scant weight to what surgical residents carried on rounds. Every morning the chief resident asked me to add a clip-art picture reflecting a recent trauma. I used the search engine AltaVista to find pictures of flipped ATVs, discharged firearms, and jackknifed trailer trucks and control+V'ed them onto the rounds sheets. The team had injuries to mend, rounds to make, and distances to maintain. The pictorial humor kept them distant enough to care for the ill and to do so quickly, on morning after morning, as they rounded past the maimed and the mutilated.

Then the trauma pager would emit a tinny, attention-piercing sound, announcing that fate was bringing another trauma case to our threshold. The team would rush to the hospital's trauma bays and take their marks. The third-year medical student waited on the periphery for their moment as the team worked through its primary survey of a body.

The trauma fellows: Airway? Protect it.

The anesthesiology residents: Breathing? Maintain it.

The medicine interns: Circulation? Control it.

The med student (*me*): Disability? Assess it.

In other words, the residents rolled a body on its side, cervical spine protected and airway secured, while I opened a pair of sterile gloves, size seven and a half, with my left hand and fished a Hemoccult card and a bottle of lube from the pockets of my short white coat with my right hand. Glove the right hand, lube it with the left, and hold the Hemoccult card open in the left. When the team signaled, I inserted a gloved and lubed index finger into the rectum and felt its muscular tone, before removing my soiled digit and smearing its sample across the card, which would reveal the presence of any blood. It was a simple test for spinal cord injuries and a simpler way to learn my place on the team. Afterward: a quick disposal of the befouled glove, a fluid-removing handwashing, and a realization that I would be a different kind of physician.

I never saw the patients I examined so invasively again. It helped maintain the clinical distance, but it demolished my own dreams.

I began the rotation dreaming of becoming a trauma surgeon because the work seemed both dramatic and necessary. It was both. I marveled at the ways patients fell apart and the ways surgeons could put them back together. The surgeons knew the body well enough to recognize its parts even when torn or crushed. While admiring their ability and their bravery, I found myself gravitating toward the older trauma surgeons, who confided that they had grown less interested in the trauma bay and the operating room and more interested in how they could prevent someone from arriving there in the first place. They wanted to know where someone lived, what they ate, how they supported themselves, whom they could confide in, whom they worshipped, and how it affected their health. They had seen enough patients on their worst days to know that what often determined a person's long-term health were the ordinary days—the day you drank again or finally got sober, the day you went hungry or were fed, the day you added to your daily walk record or decided to give up exercise—that slowly added up to an emergency.

My days were composed, like those of most med students, of intimate emergencies. I rotated off the surgery service and onto a pathological tour of all the ways our bodies fail us—a week here of pediatric neurology isolating seizure foci in anxious adolescents, two weeks there on thoracic surgery resecting cancerous lung lobes, three weeks over there of gynecological oncology debriding open abdominal wounds with a pair of tweezers and a medical-grade X-Acto knife, and then everywhere in between. I moved around the state, from hospital to hospital, so I could learn the body.

I lived along the way, asking a classmate on a date, then for her hand, which I held as she gave birth to our first child well before graduation. At home and at the hospital, we were exposed to all the fluids the body offers. An infant's stool stained our blankets. An infected person's blood was needled into my wife. A toddler's drool dampened all his clothes. A patient's tears fell on our white-coated shoulders. It was these fluids, as well as the stories we told ourselves while being exposed to them, that shaped my dreams.

I would become a psychiatrist, with fewer fluids but the most remarkable stories. To get there, I would go through a bureaucratic sorting of physicians called the Match, where a graduating medical student's choices are paired with the choices of residency programs seeking trainees. The resident physician Match sorted me to my room within the house of medicine. No more operating rooms; I spent the four years of psychiatry residency learning to ask people invasive questions in hospital and therapy rooms about how their everyday experiences added up to their emergencies. The training structured my days and nights, my thoughts and behaviors, the very way I live in the world.

. . .

In a recent year, some 150,000 premed students in the country set out on the same path. Some 62,443 people applied to an average of sixteen American medical schools. A sum of 22,666 first-year medical students, 12,590 of them women, matriculated. They joined the American physician supply chain, with its 95,475 students, 139,848 residents, and 938,966 active physicians [1]. Most of those physicians trained, like me, on a single textbook, the textbook of the body.

Today's students enter medical school as a series of metaphorical epidemics—burnout, despair, loneliness, obesity, opiates, suicide—have overlapped with a years-long pandemic. Each revealed how the inequalities in whom we train, whom we care for, and what treatments we receive have become rooted in our communities. Health is another inequality. Our whole health care system is costly; our hospitals are organized for profit rather than care; and our health insurance offers something far from universal assurance of care. Many aspiring doctors know this—just like those older trauma surgeons—and want to find ways to help.

Yet to enter medical school and to become a physician today is to have your allegiances pulled in a dozen different directions before a patient ever graces you by calling you Doctor. The obsessive focus on memorizing the body's parts and pathways repels many would-be physicians from the profession. Others enter only to feel trapped along the way—by dehumanizing environments, massive debt, or punishing hours. These flaws aren't lost on faculty, or even the medical schools that employ them, but fixing them in any meaningful way has proven impossible within the interlocking health care systems in which we all—patients, students, and physicians alike—find ourselves trapped.

Ask a practicing physician if you should go to medical school and, as often as not, they will tell you they feel trapped too. It's been bad and it's getting worse, they say, and you should not go.

They're right. No one should go to med school. It's not what you imagine. It's not what most people imagine. Many med students apply to satisfy an encouraging parent or teacher. You won't see your old teacher or even your parents for long stretches of the training. Many med students have seen glamorous portrayals of doctoring. You won't flirt with attractive colleagues nearly as often as you disimpact bowels. Many med students write admission essays about how they like science and want to help people. You can find other ways to study and serve. Many med students have heard how lucrative the work of doctoring can be. You may borrow hundreds of thousands of dollars before you finish med school and finally pay off your debt only after your hair has grayed or, like mine, fled.

So don't go. Don't go because your parents want you to be a physician. Don't go because you entertain glamorous fantasies. Don't even go because you like science. And certainly, don't go for the money.

Pursue medicine if you cannot imagine doing anything else. Study medicine because you want to understand someone else's body and community. Train as a doctor to become a physician who cares for the ill so well that they will achieve health they could not achieve without you. And if you pursue medicine, learn from two textbooks.

. . .

In this book I tell a story of a group of medical students becoming that kind of physician. It's a version of medical education and training that makes it easier for trainees to become the good physicians they wanted to become, so they can simultaneously patch up wounded bodies and improve the health of wounded communities, while personally flourishing.

The story began a few years ago when my hospital asked for someone to assess its education programs. I raised my hand. By that point in my career, I was teaching a little bit, mostly within my own specialty. The Match had sorted me, so I spent most of my time with other psychiatrists, tending to the parts of the body and mind that we were trained to see. To meet other physician educators, I started keeping office hours in the hospital's basement café. I sat and listened to anyone who would tell me about their program and their learners.

Those who talked to me astonished me with the number and variety of their learners. Piecing it all together, I figured there were more students than physicians on campus most days. I learned that students spend disproportionately large amounts of their training in safety-net systems like ours because we need them here—hospitals like mine run on thin staffing models and thinner capital margins—but also because the patients will permit students and other trainees to do more [2, 3]. Educators angered me with stories about being asked by schools if they could send us more learners because the patients at their own facilities—always wealthier and better insured—did not want to be seen by trainees. *Your patients*, they said, *are still willing to be seen by trainees.*

Listening to them, I came to understand this as the tourist model of medical education. *Come for a season and see pathology you have only read about in textbooks. Be the first person in the room when it is time to perform an invasive procedure that you read about in a journal.* Medical tourists then return home, reporting, *I loved training there. I saw so much. I got to do so much.* It is community service more than service learning.

I listened further, searching for the citizen model of medical education. *Come for a life and see patients as a fellow community member. Be the first person in the room who knows them.*

I heard it from an internist named Dr. Jennifer Adams. Listening to her story, I realized that we had lived parallel lives, both of us growing up in Colorado, heading east for college, and returning home for medicine, but she wanted to transform our shared training away from the *see one, do one, teach one* model. She sent me articles, invited me to lectures, and asked me to teach one of her students. She wanted me to know more.

When I was ready to learn more, I asked Adams if I could follow a group of her students. She quickly agreed. For five years I followed Adams and her fellow educators as they recruited, selected, trained, and graduated a cohort of medical students. I interviewed each of the students individually, recording our interviews with their permission. I observed students in clinical and educational settings, where I wrote notes in real time, eventually editing the notes for clarity and length. I worked with hundreds of medical students while preparing this story. I am grateful to them all, but especially to the students and faculty named in this book, who gave their permission and reviewed the text before publication.

To a person, med students and faculty say that their patients are their best teachers. Patients' stories are the most vital stories, but I worried about telling tales about the ill. Throughout the book, whenever a person's first and last names are used initially, they either are a public figure or gave permission to be named. When a person is first identified only by a first name, as is the case for any named patients, the name is an alias, and I altered identifying details to preserve their anonymity.

The students and the faculty are real, I assure you; so is their effort to transform medicine.

It's simple really. Instead of following physicians, medical students can follow patients. Visit patients in their homes and then accompany them on any medical encounters—primary care appointments, emergency room visits, even surgical procedures. The patient is paired with the same student the whole time, and the student gets to know the patient and where they are from. Call it a textbook-of-the-community approach, where students know patients better and serve them better. They are more focused on patients. They learn more. The experiment aims to train tomorrow's physicians today. It has one of those technical names favored by physicians, the longitudinal integrated clerkship (LIC), but everyone sounds out its acronym, L-I-C, so that it rhymes with "*Now, I see.*" *Longitudinal* is doctor talk for following patients over time. *Integrated* is doctor talk for following patients into whatever clinical setting they seek care. It's a better way of seeing patients, closer to how we all live when we are sick. This is a story of seven students learning to see patients that way, by following them wherever they go for health care, and of their faculty, who are trying to train an entire state's medical students to follow and see patients this well too.

For most of the students, entering the hospital as a third-year medical student required a narrowing of their lives, so they could participate in the drama of their patient's lives. I watched as they entered the strange-making world of the hospital for all their firsts. First patients, first births, first deaths—all helped them figure out their life's work as physicians.

But the students also lived their own lives. They struggled toward answers to the questions med students ask: How can I help other people? How can I pass the gauntlet of tests? How can I afford all the schooling? Then, how will the training change me? Can I survive the burnout, the stress, the emotional toll—and still hold on to what made me want to be a physician in the first place? Can I live my own life while helping others live theirs?

This is a story of just one program—one small group of future physicians mounting a modest insurrection within the immodest trillion-dollar health care industry—but their struggle to answer these questions, while simultaneously learning the body and the community, offers a different future for medicine. All of us—patients, physicians, students, and citizens alike—need their answer to how physicians can see patients better. We need to know what tomorrow's medicine will be. We need it to arrive soon, because the medicine of the past is killing us.

Chapter 1

DEAD *ITS*

*M*EGAN KALATA is the first of the students to meet her second dead patient. She's on trauma surgery, just a few weeks into her clinical year.

The trauma pager goes off—*GSW* [gunshot wound] *to the head ETA five minutes*. Megan, a petite woman in her twenties who clips her shoulder-length brown hair in place, races with her team to the emergency department. In transit, the surgery resident preps her, in a shorthand fashion. "Just so you know, people who have gunshot wounds to the head generally don't survive."

Duly warned, Megan arrives at the trauma bay as it fills with more than a dozen people. The room smells of latex gloves, industrial cleaning supplies, and the sweat pearling up on the clinicians despite the odorless air conditioning.

Megan moves away, huddled together with a classmate in an out-of-the-way corner of the room to watch the teamwork. A bullet's entry point requires little skill to observe, but the skilled people in the room know the distinctive destructive paths different kinds of bullets carve inside the cranium. They know how to work determinedly, and together, to stop bleeding and prevent further damage to the brain. The hospital has a reputation as one of the best and fastest trauma centers in the country, but this time, the team is moving with less speed than expected. Watching the half-speed clinical bustle of the trauma team, Megan catches a peculiar energy. The clinicians are behaving, she senses, as if their work will soon be over.

Confirming that hunch, the team calls the students up, like rookies off the bench to finish off a rout, to stand at the center table. Her friend does a full two minutes, then Megan takes over the compressions. Megan's resting expression is a smile that involves her whole face, while masking her resolute determination. Megan places the heel of one hand over the sternum and interlaces the fingers of her other hand to keep them off the patient's chest. Then she presses down and up, down and up, worrying about whether she is doing it right.

A resident reassures her. "If the table is too high and you're too short, or if you get tired, step out of the way and I'll take over."

A nurse helps her keep time. "Okay. Go, go, go."

She feels bolstered by the staff's encouragement, even as doubts creep in.

"I don't know how time works when you're doing that," Megan said, "but after thirty seconds or a minute, that was when they stopped everything and said, 'Okay, we're going to check one more time for a pulse,' and asked if anyone could think of anything else they could do differently."

Megan is the last person to attempt resuscitation, the last person to lay hands on the patient before he becomes, through a physician's declaration, a corpse.

"I think as a med student, in the back of your mind, you know that no one's ever going to really let you do anything bad or wrong, but you're also nervous. Whatever you're doing, whether it's closing a patient's skin or doing chest compressions, you have this thought of 'Who decided I could do this? Who let me in here to do this?' But also: 'I really want to be here doing it and I want to do a good job with whatever *it* is.'"

That day, the *it* was practicing CPR on a patient in his final moments.

Afterward, as the nurses clean up and the resident physicians file paperwork, Megan speaks with her classmate. They both noticed the same thing.

"The patient had a gunshot wound to the head, but he also had a gunshot wound to the hand that was through and through. I had been thinking, what were those last moments like for him? Was his hand up by his head? Was there one gunshot or two gunshots? But either way, no one was paying attention to the patient's hand, and the hand was laying over the side of the bed with blood pouring out of it. And I got blood on my scrubs because it was just pouring out of the hand and because it was not something that anybody was caring about when this person had this gunshot wound to his head."

The bleeding hand was not the *it*. The blood on Megan's hand was not the *it*. The violent death of the patient—the heartache it would bring, the generations it would fracture—was not the *it*.

"I didn't feel as sad as I would have thought that I would when seeing someone die. Then I felt kind of guilty for not feeling sad about it. But I didn't know this person. I never saw them, never talked to them, didn't see this person open their eyes."

Megan learned how you can maintain emotional distance while gaining clinical skills on a dying person, even as he bleeds on you from a hole in his hand where a bullet passed through.

. . .

Maintaining emotional distance is one of the central lessons of medical training. For at least the past century, we have taught it before any other lesson. When the sociologist Frederic Hafferty observed medical training, he found that the first lessons of medical school occurred in the cadaver lab. A student's first assigned patient, Hafferty observed, was a cadaver, and it socialized the student to the doctor's role. That dead patient was also the patient with whom she would spend the most time for her entire career, the patient she would know best. But what would the student know? Not their hopes, their failures, or sorrows like those of a friend. Not even their name, their rank, or their identifying number like a prisoner of war. A student would open a body and leaf through it to see how it resembled an anatomy atlas. Students learned to locate problems within individual people, explicitly the patient, but implicitly in themselves. Medical culture, Hafferty wrote, implicitly encourages students to "locate the source of their troubles in their own personalities rather than in the structure of the educational experience" [4, p. 17]. Medical schools use psychological language, which students adopt, to describe their enculturation as an internal reality (what they feel and think), rather than an external one (what they do and how they spend their time). A student's minutes, hours, days, weeks, and months became subsumed into medical time in windowless cadaver labs before they learned to subsume their lives into the hospital. By the end of the lab time, a student dismantled her cadaver into her first textbook and built herself into someone who could focus on the skills necessary to resuscitate a trauma victim even while he was becoming a corpse underneath her hands. Medical education changed her into the kind of person who, after breaking open the body like a favorite text, will later perform invasive exams, become dirtied by its bodily fluids, and yet maintain emotional distance. That is what medicine has wanted from physicians for the past hundred years, to know the failing body intimately, to face death directly, all while retaining clinical equanimity.

. . .

We gain from equanimity—the composure and even temper—when a physician prioritizes a patient's needs above her own in difficult situations. We lose from equanimity when a physician is so composed that she becomes distant from her own interior life, the people in her life, and the people she meets as patients. Dosing medical students with the right amount of equanimity is the challenge for medical schools: enough for a student to respond to a trauma, not so much that they become traumatized by the work. And the places that deliver medical school's strongest doses are the cadaver lab and the trauma bay, the places where a sick person becomes an *it*, where a person becomes a textbook that can be seen, done, taught. This is the textbook of the body.

Occasionally, though, a student finds herself in one of those places and personhood intrudes, and she needs to know more, needs to be something more than merely composed.

Not long after seeing her second dead person, Megan was called to see what would have been, in an earlier medical era, her third dead person.

A bad car accident brought five people into the hospital. Megan was assigned to the person most grievously injured. The team spent six hours with the patient in the operating room, and Megan says, "It was touch and go with her for a long time." Trauma surgeons can save people who surely would have died only a few years ago, and in this case, after all their overnight effort, the patient survived. Megan recounts that as she was finally leaving at the end of her shift that morning, "we walked past the SICU waiting area, and there were maybe thirty-five or forty people, all sitting there, all there for her, and crying and praying and talking to each other."

It hit her. All night, she was with their loved one, on the same floor, separated by one corridor and her clinical distance. As she closed the physical gap, the clinical distance collapsed as well. She wanted to go to them, comfort them somehow. But the rest of the surgical team was headed out the door in search of scant sleep.

Megan recognized their response as professionally sound: they saw it many times before, and they would see it many times again, so they blocked it out to stay emotionally steady. Emergency physicians and surgeons talked about their work's shifting "D/B," or death-to-beauty ratio, and admitted that getting on the wrong side of the ratio could pull a physician down. Megan followed the team out the door.

For most med students, that would be the story's end. The patient would remain an *it* they encountered during trauma, whose family keeping vigil they would walk silently past.

But Megan is different, so it was the story's beginning. The patient survived the night, and Megan added her to her list of longitudinal patients. She learned the patient's name: Esmeralda. As Megan followed Esmeralda through her stay in the hospital, Esmeralda became visible to her, familiar, known. She knew Esmeralda across time, how she lived, whom she loved, whom she worshiped. The textbook of the community.

When Megan compares her response to those two trauma patients, she names the felt difference between mourning a person and mourning an *it*.

"I felt a lot more emotion with her because we were there with her all night and saw her family crying. Then she was a patient that my team kept following, so we were checking on her every day, and then I met some of her family members and learned more about her. She is a single mom and has two kids."

The clinical year transforms every medical student into a particular kind of physician. How it changes you depends on how you learn to work with other people. Pathologists see death's premonitions in tissue samples. Trauma surgeons tragically feel death take over a body under their hands. Primary care practitioners attend to a person who slowly sickens and dies. Medical students decide what relationship they desire with death, an uncommon decision for people their age. They need to know the body, but they can also know more. Knowing more about Esmeralda impacted Megan's response. Megan saw her as a mother. Then she thought about the victim, nameless to her, with the fatal gunshot piercing his head and hand.

"I felt kind of guilty not having that same emotion for that other person. So, yeah, guilty." Megan wanted to transmute that guilt into a resolution, to be the kind of physician who knew the body well but could also be close enough to her patients that she could know them as people, even share some of their emotions. She wasn't quite sure what kind of physician training she would seek in the Match, which assigns doctors to a specialty. Since Megan wanted to know her patients and be known by her patients, she was learning from a physician who had found a way to teach students from two textbooks: the textbook of the body and the textbook of the community.

Chapter 2

PUNISHER TIME

$\mathcal{D}$R. JENNIFER ADAMS finds her old nemesis waiting behind the exam room door. Her quick brown eyes scan the clinical triangle: computer, clock, table. The computer sits on a worktable with a recessed sink where she performs ablutions with scalding water and antimicrobial soap. The clock above the sink sweeps away the seconds into minutes, hours, and days. The patient sits, eyes down and shoulders slumped, on an examination table that fills the middle of the crowded room, like a throne relocated to a closet. Adams sits in a work chair, swiveling between the computer and the examination table, where Lorenzo catches her up quickly.

"I was doing well, then I went down south. I was training. Then my privates started swelling. They had to do surgery." With his right hand, he scoops his testicles through his sweatpants and says, "There were a couple of infections in there."

At his report, Adams drops the corners of her mouth into a disapproving frown, tilts her head, and scrunches her shoulders, underneath her long layered brown hair, backward in concern. "Oh Lorenzo, I heard about this. I'm so sorry."

Lorenzo lifts his dark eyes, brimming with tears, up to meet hers.

The clock ticks off a pair of seconds. Adams brings her head back to the vertical and begins talking, moving fluidly between the language of personal concern and that of impersonal science. "I saw that you were hospitalized for two weeks with an abscess in your seminal vesicles. Your health has been such a seesaw. You have your chronic conditions. Arthritis, diabetes. If I prescribe medications to suppress your immune system, it will make those better. Your inflammation will be reduced, you'll feel less pain, and be able to train. But it will also predispose you to infections."

Lorenzo releases his swollen testicles and slumps resignedly as she recounts the illnesses narrowing his life. He has lived all his fifty-something years in Colorado. Many of his loved ones and their sentinel events—sudden deaths, devastating illness—are commemorated in the multiple colorless tattoos decorating his arms. Some of the tattoos are partially covered by his black T-shirt, which advertises a local boxing camp. Lorenzo promotes fights. When well, Lorenzo fights his own fights.

Today, Lorenzo needs Adams to fight for him. He watches her face, breaking eye contact only to look over her shoulder at the computer displaying surgical reports. Adams catches his peering eyes, pivots the computer's monitor toward him, and clicks on a list of his medications—*colchicine, diclofenac, etanercept, ferrous sulfate, insulin, metformin, miconazole, omeprazole, oxycodone, prednisone, sertraline.* Adams reviews each medication and asks Lorenzo to repeat their names back to her, like a navigator repeating the starry landmarks directing a sailor on his journey.

Reassured by his familiarity, Adams clicks over to the health record's problem list. The list is numbered and hierarchical, with the most pressing concerns first. She starts at the top and, for each problem, addresses Lorenzo's current state and the obstacles to treatment. Surgery to repair his hernia is dangerous. Medication to control his arthritis is beyond his means.

Working through the problem list, Adams draws Lorenzo toward her with her concern. When he surprises her with an answer, her easy laugh warms the exam room. When he expresses despair, her consoling hands reassure him quickly. While Lorenzo sits, she fidgets, fiddling with the stethoscope around her neck, lifting her toes to rock her sockless feet onto her heels, and raising her arm to catch the time. She winces and interrupts Lorenzo.

"How is your diabetes?"

"My blood sugar got to 40 one day."

"What happened?"

"I forgot to eat."

"Ohhh, Enzo, you can't forget. When you're on insulin, eating consistently is as important as taking the medication the right way. You've got to call me. Call me directly with questions. I'm sorry you got that low. I don't like that for you."

He nods agreement.

Adams offers Lorenzo her arm to steady him into position for the physical exam. She unwraps the dusty Ace bandage constraining his swollen right wrist and then washes her hands in the sink. While rinsing, she engages Lorenzo's silent seven-year-old grandson.

"And how are you?"

"I'm starting to train too, to spar."

"Oh." Adams raises an eyebrow. "Why aren't you in school today?"

Lorenzo answers for his grandson, "I need to take him to fill out some paperwork so he can stay with me."

Adams nods and files her concern for the grandson away for another day. She unties Lorenzo's shoes, removes his socks, and examines his swollen joints. Then she turns Lorenzo's face away from hers, draws the fingers of her left hand into a fist, and pounds his kidneys.

"You're used to sparring in the ring. How does it feel to spar with a doctor?"

Lorenzo groans at the medical humor, but Adams is undaunted, continuing her examination and her therapeutic cajoling.

"When your sugar is out of control, the bacteria in your urine just has a feast, so we've got to get your sugars under control."

Lorenzo nods again.

Adams steps toward the sink to wash her hands again. Lorenzo rewraps his right wrist with a bandage. Adams has a plan. She will order blood work, urinalysis, and an ophthalmology exam to track the progress of his disease. Lorenzo will sign forms to release more records from his recent hospitalization. She will update his eleven medications in the computer to secure refills and call his insurance company to plead for access to a new medication. He will return home as a patient—no boxing while ill. She flicks off the faucet with her wrist.

Adams accelerates out of the crowded room. Striding down the hallway, she collects Lorenzo's prescriptions from a printer and scribbles her signature. She asks her medical assistant to deliver the signed scripts to Lorenzo, schedule him for a return appointment, and print out coloring pages for his grandson.

Adams ducks into the physician workroom, a galley room perpendicular to the clinic's hallway, and slides into an empty chair. Logging on to a computer, her schedule appears and an alarm pops up. Crystal, a new patient with an urgent concern, has been added to her already full afternoon. The patient is late, so Adams waits, doomscrolling through the emails on her computer and the text messages on her phone. Before she sounds their depths, she bolts up from her chair. "I forgot to talk to him about the plan for the rectal tumor we found on a screening colonoscopy." She strides down the hallway and tells Lorenzo about the tumor. She counsels deferring the exam until his current crises are resolved. Lorenzo agrees, thanks her for remembering, and says goodbye. As Adams moves down the hallway, faster now, Lorenzo shuffles out. The back of his boxing T-shirt declares, in block white letters above a pair of boxing gloves, "IT'S PUNISHER TIME!"

...

The timekeepers—the clock on the wall, the computer on the desk, the watch on her wrist, and the phone in her pocket—punish a primary care physician like Adams. The clinic manager tracking the minutes she spends with patients. The clinic coder translating those minutes into the bills that keep the clinic open. The patients visiting her in clinic once a month, once a quarter, or once a crisis occurs. The patients often arrive late for appointments, reducing their time to get at the root of crises. The visits are scheduled for fifteen minutes, during which she is attending a person whose daily life diverges from hers in every detail— where they sleep, what they eat, how they move, what labor they undertake, whom they love, and how they worship. She has fifteen minutes to address the fact that her patients are literally losing time, dying decades younger than people who live in wealthier, whiter neighborhoods of Denver.

The interstate highways intersect just north of downtown Denver, bringing commerce and trade from across the nation, while marking out opportunities for health and wealth. Denver is organized around I-25, which runs south from Las Cruces, New Mexico, and north to Buffalo, Wyoming, and I-70, which runs from Cove Fort, Utah, to Baltimore, Maryland. The Inverted L, the area south of I-70 and east of I-25, prospers in every way. Most of the city's best hospitals, neighborhoods, and schools are within the Inverted L, while most of the city's polluting factories and waste facilities are outside the Inverted L. If you live within the Inverted L, you are more likely to be white, educated, and wealthy, and to have trees in your front yard.

Adams, like most of the city's physicians, lives inside the Inverted L, and she has the front-yard trees to show for it. Unlike most of the city's physicians, Adams works where diseases and disabilities concentrate, outside the Inverted L. She commutes from her own neighborhood to a pair of federally qualified health centers (FQHCs). At one FQHC, Adams sees persons with HIV. At the other, she meets Lorenzo. This FQHC, located on a bus line on the city's west side, has a pharmacy and a laboratory to minimize a patient's health travels, as well as social workers and outreach workers to secure additional health resources. Dentists and obstetricians are on the first floor, pediatricians and internists on the second floor. Adams is an internist, and for each half day she works at the FQHC she sees ten patients on the second floor in limited windows of time. She uses the time to teach: how to take medications, how ailments affect health, and how to receive more services. She teaches patients like Lorenzo to name and know their bodies, in sickness and in health. She also teaches medical students and residents to spend enough time with patients—a decade's worth of students have followed Lorenzo with her—so they, too, have something to offer them.

So as Adams enters the workroom again to document her encounter with Lorenzo, an internal medicine resident interrupts her to discuss a patient with a mysterious illness. The patient reportedly has tinea capitis, a fungal infection that feeds off the fibrous proteins in hair, but it has not responded to the usual curative treatments for tinea. The resident wonders if the diagnosis is wrong and displays pictures that look like crop circles cut in the hair behind the patient's ears and on the top of her head. As Adams reviews the photos, her voice rises enthusiastically at pathophysiological possibilities. *Contact dermatitis. Lupus. Tumors. Battle's sign.* Her enthusiasm elicits other physicians in the room, who stand up from their workstations to look at the pictures and offer alternative diagnoses. Adams leads the conversation, encouraging the resident to consult dermatology and publish a case report. Then she catches the time and ends the conversation. The gathered physicians retreat from pictures of mysterious pathology to the quotidian work of primary care.

They call their room the bullpen. The seats are unreserved, with physicians sitting at whichever of the six workstations are available. Between patient visits, the physicians log in and lock on to their computer screens, reviewing patient charts, documenting encounters, and looking up phone numbers to call patients with reports of lab tests and imaging studies. The room smells faintly of the half-eaten lunches moldering next to workstations. The steady sounds in the room are fingers tapping on the electronic keyboards, argon gas humming within fluorescent ceiling lights, and the spinning of fans within computers.

The fans keep the computers from overheating as the physicians type every finding into Epic, the cloud-based electronic health record (EHR) that the hospital employs. There are so many visits to summarize, prescriptions to sign, and queries to answer that many of the physicians spend most of their workday—and too many evenings—charting. Specialty physicians often earn enough to hire scribes who accompany them and complete their documentation chores. Primary care physicians typically earn a fraction of that salary, so they spend more time tending the EHR than other physicians. Between them, this group has decades of clinical experience and over a hundred years of schooling, but they are spending their afternoon in data entry.

Whether it is the data entry, the ever-changing medical knowledge they must keep up with, the comparatively lower pay of primary care physicians, or the difficulty of doctoring patients whose social problems determine their health, fewer and fewer medical students are choosing this work. And even as fewer new physicians commit to primary care, others leave the profession early. Adams is staying in the field—for now. She is, on most days, surviving medicine. She uses time purposefully, to see patients who are invisible to most physicians and to train a generation of physicians to follow her into the work. She is creating an education program that teaches an entire state's physicians to turn their shared nemesis—time—into their tool. She hopes it will eventually transform medicine.

. . .

For now, time is against her. Crystal, the twenty-one-year-old added to her schedule, arrives late. Adams heads out of the bullpen and into the exam room. Crystal has a cold, which should not take long. But Adams and Crystal are strangers to each other, so Adams needs a brief history. Her questions yield the predicted diagnosis—an upper respiratory infection (URI)—and Adams recommends supportive treatment and a flu shot. Adams behaves as if the encounter is over, but Crystal pulls her smartphone out and asks if she could show "one more thing" to the doctor. Crystal swipes through pictures of mosquito bites on her legs sustained during a vacation. Adams asks a few questions, reassures Crystal that these are simple mosquito bites, and tries (again) to conclude the encounter. Crystal parries with headaches. Adams queries and diagnoses tension headaches. Crystal agrees, then adds anxiety. Adams searches for closure.

"We're running low on time today, but at your next visit I want to explore your anxiety, because that's a treatable condition."

"I've been wanting to talk about that for a while, but I've been saving things up to talk to a doctor. I'm anxious all the time. I have mood swings. I get angry. I make fists. My knuckles aren't happy with the way I feel." Crystal thrusts the dorsal surface of her hands into the space between her and Adams. "See, all the skin is off my hands." Adams examines Crystal's knuckles, reassuring herself that while Crystal's anxiety may run deep, these abrasions are superficial. Adams politely defers further questions.

Crystal is undeterred. "I am also having lady problems." Adams takes another five minutes to review the sights and smells of vaginal discharges, both infectious and normal.

When Adams finally leaves the room, after forty minutes with a patient who arrived fifteen minutes late for a fifteen-minute add-on visit, she has already missed the marks for her afternoon schedule. Crystal, like many patients, has more ailments than allotted time. It is probably clinically ideal for Adams to see only fifteen patients a day, but this is what society offers Crystal, a circumscribed visit with a primary care physician in which they work together through a tangled list of mental, physical, and social problems, seeking some version of hope [5].

Back in the workroom, Adams chides herself. "That was painful. I thought it was going to be a simple URI, and then she had a list. One of my fellow internists, Dr. Josh Blum, has a saying, 'Seize the list,' and I've embraced that. Today, I didn't seize the list. The list seized me and I paid for it." Blum's aphorism, *carpe album*, is a riff on Horace's ode on living with time, his ancient admonition to "prune back your long-term hopes. Life ebbs as I speak—so seize each day" [6, p. 79]. To seize the clinical day, to master the envious moment, you must prune hopes and seize the problem list before it seizes you.

She tries again. Preparing for her next patient, she says, "If I set up the note beforehand, everything goes better. I'm just cutting and pasting a bit." Adams reviews the notes from her next patient's last visit and builds a skeleton note for today's encounter, drawing forward the problem list, medications, and treatment plans for Wanda, a woman in her fifties.

Her note prepped, Adams enters the exam room to find Wanda waiting.

"How are you doing?" Adams asks, taking a seat as she, again, logs on to the exam room's workstation.

"Not good, not good. I'm in pain all the time, just throwing up at work."

"Oooh, I'm so sorry. Well, once I get my computer to start, I want to review the results of your endoscopy." Together they review Wanda's

gradual entry to the kingdom of the sick. Months ago, Wanda com-
plained of gastrointestinal distress. Adams responded with a referral to a
specialist, one of the defensive strategies of the time-burdened primary
care physician [5]. The gastroenterologists observed too much inflammation to make a clear diagnosis. Adams changed Wanda's medications,
added omeprazole, and ordered a repeat biopsy, hoping for a definitive
diagnosis. For now, she stalls, because while she suspects that Wanda
has cancer, she is still waiting for the pathology report. "Our hope, our
very much hope, is that if it is an ulcer from the common causes, the
omeprazole will treat it. If it's not, then the biopsy will tell us that it's cancer. It worries me that this is still causing you pain. I'm concerned."

Cancer. Tears form at the corners of Wanda's eyes.

Adams reassures her by relaying what she heard from the gastroenterologist. "She called me when you were asleep and said 'I'm worried.
It doesn't look good.' But then she called me after the biopsies and said,
'The biopsies came back negative.' That encourages me. She's a great
doctor and you're in good hands. But I don't want to give you any false
hopes."

Wanda nods at the small hope Adams holds out, that the determi-
native biopsy will be benign, and the larger hope Adams represents,
an honest answer and a caring presence. They are both striving toward
a future for Wanda that they cannot be sure will exist. They discuss
her other symptoms and plans for treatment until her next endoscopy
in two weeks. The dates are specific; the hopes are vague.

"I just hope for the best."

"We do too. I will say that if it is a gastric cancer, we'll treat it aggressively. I'm here for you. We'd have our oncology team and likely
our surgery team. The good news is this just started a few months ago.
If it's cancer, we'll move quick. I'll be here every step of the way."

Adams reviews the eleven medications she prescribes for Wanda, as
well as the over-the-counter medications Wanda prescribes herself,

and then lowers the lever of the examination table. She looks at Wanda's abdomen, then listens and touches. Adams frowns as she asks about foods Wanda can tolerate. When Wanda settles on yogurt, Adams smiles.

"Forget everything you learned about eating vegetables and lean meats. I want you to eat anything smooth that is appetizing. I don't want you to lose any more weight. If your appetite is poor and your stomach is filling up, I want you to get the protein and vegetables you can tolerate, but mostly I want you to eat what you can tolerate. A milkshake may be the best medicine."

Adams and Wanda have a treatment plan. And Adams has even made up a bit of the time she lost to Crystal. Then, as the conscientious Adams often does, she gives the time up. No *carpe album* today.

"Can I bring up one other thing? I'm really worried about your smoking. I know it's hard to think about quitting right now, but I worry that every time you light up a cigarette, it irritates your ulcer. You need to quit. What can I do to help you?"

Wanda looks Adams square in the eyes, settling on whom and what to hope for and what to ask for. She looks as if she will demand a clear answer today—cancer or no—but she eventually responds to the question.

"Dr. Adams, I just need to quit. I know about addiction, and I know I have to stop."

Adams nods. "Remember, any time is a good time to quit." Wanda demurs, so Adams concludes the visit with a summary of next steps and a final invitation. "I want you to have a notebook where you write down questions and worries. Then can I give you a call at the end of the week so that I can answer your questions? Then we'll have you back in a few weeks to get the results of your repeat endoscopy, review them together, and then cross whatever bridge is ahead of you."

Wanda thanks her, promises to write, and falls silent.

Adams prepares to leave, but Wanda's hopes have flagged. She asks, softly now, "Why didn't someone find this sooner?"

. . .

Afterward, back in the workroom, the question is still bothering Adams. "I thought Dr. __ had told her about the cancer. I would have scheduled a double appointment if I knew I had to tell her she had cancer."

The digital clocks around Adams rely on counting the ticktock of a fixed frequency and measure the oscillations against standard units. The internal clocks of patients rely on feeling the ticktock of shifting frequencies, of when it is time to quit cigarettes, of when it is time to drink milkshakes. Human clocks count expectations, whether the speed of an encounter or the words of a physician.

Human time stretches in response to our expectations, and no expectations are more profound than those in which people place their hopes. Hope cannot be measured in standard units like minutes and hours and days. For a physician, hope is not an emotion. Hope is not wishful thinking because you see how often people sicken and die. Hope is not a stoic fearlessness in the face of adversity. Hope is not a Spartan endurance through a losing battle against an insurmountable foe. Hope is what a physician offers to a patient so they can survive today's crisis, while striving toward a tomorrow. Hope is a practice.

A good physician doubles time when she dashes hope. Cancer takes longer to tell because it forecloses futures. Instead of longevity, the cancer patient hopes a doctor can relieve symptoms or that a surgeon can induce a five-year survival rate. The cancer patient's hopes are immediate and pragmatic, well sized for receiving medical care, for this day's surgery, this hour's medications, this moment's assessment. There's no time but today. Seize it. Order the milkshake.

A good physician halves time when she encourages hope. Cure takes little time to tell because it reopens futures. Instead of spending time shuttling between clinics, the cured patient hopes to leave the regular care of physicians and be a patient no more. The cured person's hopes are expansive and transcendent, well sized for living with others, for this day's labors, next month's plans, the decades ahead.

Adams scheduled the wrong amount of time for Wanda, because she thought the gastroenterologist had already foreclosed some of Wanda's hopes. All Adams can do is borrow time with the medical hope of a definitive diagnosis in the near future, so she returns to Wanda, reviews the plan, and asks again, "Does that sound okay?"

Wanda nods. OK. The human condition in a single word.

. . .

The most spoken word on the planet—*OK, okay, ok*—travels easily, acquiring various marks along the way: ôkê in Vietnam, oké in Hungary, and ocá in Brazil. It is malleable enough to indicate acceptance, acknowledgment, or assent, and it can live anywhere in a sentence, as an adjective, noun, or verb. The word's linguistic plasticity lends itself to the ambiguous moments that commonly occur in a medical encounter. "Okay" keeps a range of hopes open. Acceptance, acknowledgment, or assent—either way, Dr. Adams is promising to stay with Wanda. It's not hope, but it's something like it, and "okay" helps a physician move through the list.

Adams and Wanda finish the list with unspoken questions. *Who will tell the full truth? Who will help? What do I do? What do I say?* They share the existential questions that today's medicine leaves a primary care physician and a patient, both with imperfect access to the specialists who provide the definitive treatment. They make it, together, to an okay.

Everyone who knows Adams will tell you that she says okay easily but struggles to say no. As her afternoon clinic session unfurls, she says yes to every good request. Throughout the clinic session, she apologizes often for being behind the clock but keeps on saying okay to her patients. But as she assents to every good request with her time, she keeps hopes afloat. When her patients ask Adams about this spot on their limb or that ache in their belly, she answers, and her patients receive her as a hope.

Earning another okay closure, Adams returns to the workroom. This time, Catherine Ard, a young medical student who shares the same easy smile over a determined jaw, is waiting. While Adams moves with an anxious energy, Catherine calmly lopes. Catherine is back from the hospital's tumor board, an interdisciplinary conference where they discuss patients being treated with cancer. It's the kind of place at which Wanda's future care could be discussed. Experienced physicians trained in subspecialties will debate the best way—the knife, the laser, the pill—to treat a tumor. Catherine was short at least a decade of training compared to everyone else in the room but found a way to contribute to the care of one of Adams's patients. Catherine provided information she learned from following the patient over time. Catherine proudly reports to Adams that it changed the conversation and opened more treatment options. Adams has made a career of moving forward by holding on to one small detail after another until she summits a task, and she cheers the news: her student may have just secured more time, more life, for her patient.

Adams herself has seven more patients to see this afternoon, but she eagerly catches up with her student. Adams hopes Catherine will soon match into internal medicine, maybe even here, so Catherine can be the future that extends Adams's current work. Adams wants medical students like Catherine to accompany patients on visits to specialist clinics, to scrub in for patients' surgical procedures, to keep watch with patients on the wards, and to visit patients' homes to see how they implement doctors' orders. Adams is teaching Catherine to journey with patients, so they can turn time into trust and secure a little hope together.

Chapter 3

CHASED DREAMS

*T*HE STUDENTS ARE ANXIOUS to know what the future holds—the kind of physician they will become and where—and the first clues are in the gifts the faculty are bearing.

On the curved stage of a large lecture hall, the dean of the University of Colorado School of Medicine stands alongside attending and resident physicians, all with more gray hairs, wrinkles, and pounds than the fresh-faced students. The standing physicians take turns telling doctor stories, self-deprecating but also self-aggrandizing. They offer advice for the rising third-year medical students seated in the large lecture hall. *Learn always. Listen often. Sleep where you can.* It feels like parents gifting their children with advice, but no one is kin here; it's a found family.

At advice's end, the faculty and the students stand together and recite a pledge whose last lines are from the Hippocratic oath: *May I always act so as to preserve the finest traditions of my calling, and may I long experience the joy of healing those who seek my help.* The oath is the profession's promise that they will cross familial lines. They swear to apprentice themselves to the surrogate parents of the faculty. They vow to care for ill strangers as if they were family.

. . .

For Sarah Bardwell, it is a pledge that she will chase her dream all the way to its end.

Sarah Bardwell followed her dream, in every direction, working as a mechanic, nanny, and waitress before standing here as a med student. She ran anarchist bike shops, married a boyfriend to forestall his deportation, and learned to tattoo her own arms—with hearts and hobo symbols and a picture of herself on a swing, as if her arms were the trunks of a favorite tree. The through line for each tattoo—for her experiences—is the family dream. Her grandfather was a labor organizer, her mother an anti–nuclear war activist; raised on social justice, Sarah protested and marched as a child, as a student, and as an adult. She is thirty-five, one of the oldest medical students in her class, but she is becoming a physician to live out her own petitions.

She plans to do so at Denver Health. It's the place she imagines when she hears the word "hospital." As a child living nearby, its public health physicians tested her for lead exposure. It is her first memory of a medical encounter: a worried child, a negative test, a reassured parent, a positive encounter. As an adult, she moved closer, living less than a mile from the hospital for the past decade, close enough to see patients walk out carrying the pink plastic bags marked "PATIENT BE-LONGINGS" that they received at discharge. She experienced more of what it offered. She saw that it was a general hospital, meaning that it cared for people with all varieties of medical conditions, but also a safety-net hospital, meaning that it specialized in serving the varieties of the marginalized ill: the uninsured, the undocumented, the unhinged, the undesirable. Sarah always felt welcome. She accompanied many friends to its emergency department, hospital wards, and outpatient clinics. The buildings were modest, even scruffy, but the care was excellent and expansive. Denver Health is a system, running the city's paramedic, psychiatric, and public health services, while managing dozens of clinics in the city's public schools, jails, and lower-income neighborhoods; it is one of the first community health center networks in the country, and still one of the largest [7, 8]. For Sarah, it remains something simple. "If there wasn't Denver Health, there wouldn't be health care for most of the people I know and work with." She dreams of joining so she can provide health care for the people she knows. But, as of now, that dream is still over the horizon. Sarah is on the LIC wait-list, so she is slated to spend her clinical year elsewhere.

· · ·

For more than a century, medical students have followed orders and rules, standardized at the turn of the nineteenth century by reformers who remade medical education for the meritocracy. Reformers en-shrined the Puritan work ethic and the stiff lips, upper and lower; the stoic nature, in good times and bad; the self-discipline, in school and in the hospital. Generations of medical students learned the code and be-came loyal to the side of medicine, learning to show their merit badges to the house of medicine to suggest that they were made of similar stuff. Over the past hundred years the desired merits became codified. Be able-bodied. Enjoy citizenship. Attend a leading college. Graduate with the highest marks. Accrue research experience. Join the sixty-thousand-plus students who apply to an average of sixteen medical schools each year for the nation's twenty-two thousand first-year medical school positions. Enroll in the most prominent medical school that accepts you. Once there, you become one of the ninety-five thousand people enrolled in American medical schools at any given time [1]. Outscore the mean on every acronymic standardized test—SAT, MCAT, USMLE—placed before you. Honor every course. A stu-dent who successfully travels this well-demarcated route through the meritocracy keeps every path open.

The LIC program is designed to show students a different way of becoming—and practicing as—a physician. It's a curriculum that studies both the text of the community and the text of the body. And, if Dr. Jennifer Adams is right, it's an approach that can scale and spread, spurring a transformation in the way medicine is practiced for decades to come.

She started small. For the past four years, Adams has recruited eight med students from the 184 students in the second-year class. This year, there are so many interested students that Adams is determined to expand the experiment. To do so, she needs more money and more space. She schedules a meeting with hospital administrators to ask for more. The day before the meeting, she worried about whether she could endorse more dreams and welcome students like Sarah to the program. Adams wears some of her worries on her forehead as lines of experience, but these worries increased into illness. "I was so stressed. I kept on bending over, grabbing my abdomen, and joking to people, 'it must be my appendix.' I kept going, but that night, I was hosting the LIC students at my house for a dinner. I wasn't hungry, couldn't eat. As the students talked, I realized it was a textbook case—the pain started generalized, then localized to McBurney's point. I finished the evening with them and then went to the hospital. They took my appendix out and all I could think of was what I was missing. I had a big presentation to give the next day. I was going to ask for more funds for the students and there I was, sick myself."

She missed the meeting, so a friend delivered the presentation. It was good enough to secure additional funds to grow the LIC from eight students to ten. Adams receives the news from her own hospital bed; she dreams of even more students, but this will do for today. She endures a day of recovery and then returns, pain be damned, to doctoring. Less than forty-eight hours after being under the knife, she is seeing patients in her clinic and teaching students in her classroom, all while seeking students whose dedication rises to just the right level—the ones who will follow their patients even while recovering from their own ailments.

Sarah's dedication ascends, and Adams calls her off the waitlist, offering her a third-year assignment that shares her commitment to social justice based at the hospital she knows best. Sarah's next dream, of someday running a free clinic that provides medical care in neighborhoods that feel forgotten by modern advances, is a step closer. Sarah will spend her clinical year at Denver Health. After spending the two prior years memorizing every muscle and nerve, every resulting twitch that animates each breath and heartbeat, she gets to meet patients of her own. After cramming her head with the intended and adverse effects of hundreds of medicines, she gets to help prescribe. After working incessantly to earn high marks on dozens of the gatekeeping tests, she will finally understand what a real test is, what the work really entails.

Not every well-prepared med student ends up where they expected when starting the clinical year, and any number of forces can crush the dreams of Sarah and her peers. Some call the clinical year "the cynical year," because so many student dreams are soured by the structures and strictures of medicine. Burnout, debt, and overwork are common, especially as more physicians are working within larger health care systems whose celebrated virtues are efficiency, haste, and profit. The students will soon meet the routine dilemmas that become the daily bread of a physician's work, all while deciding what type of physician they want to be, or if they want to be physicians at all. This is the year when they chase their dreams until, through the Match, they realize the dream they will live out.

. . .

To prepare her students, Dr. Adams brings her new class together a few days after the oath ceremony. The text at hand? Not Hippocrates, but an orientation manual.

One of the first students to arrive is Mackenzie Garcia. From the moment she entered medical school, Mackenzie telegraphed her keen interest in the LIC. Mackenzie wears her hair short, her eyeglasses large, and her heart on her sleeve. She grew up in Evergreen, a small town on the boundary between Colorado's urban core and its mountain playgrounds, worked as a patient navigator in AmeriCorps before med school, and wants to become a primary care physician in an FQHC. She was drawn to the LIC both because of its location at a safety-net hospital and because of the way it teaches. Her hope is that the continuity of the LIC will give her a better shot at caring for patients.

As the students trickle into the orientation session, Dr. Adams warms them up by asking how they spent the small vacation between the second and third years of med school. Many traveled: Moab, Vegas, Cabo, Philly, even Denmark, seizing the chance to see a world beyond the hospital in which they will soon immerse themselves. Sarah loves hiking in state and national parks but sheepishly reports that she was so tired that she just slept in.

The students dress like college students who woke up fifteen minutes ago, not like physicians yet. The students rest large backpacks on the floor before unpacking their immediate needs onto the table before them. Out comes breakfast—yogurt, bananas, chia pudding—as Adams speaks. Water bottles or travel mugs of coffee sit within reach. One student sets a 32-ounce water bottle, a recycled pickle jar full of cold brew coffee, and a jar of gel cap ibuprofen before her. Water, coffee, and analgesics. They bring their own gifts forward as they prepare to live out the profession's oaths.

Adams begins walking students through their manual: how to park their cars, borrow scrubs, access hospital gyms, and enter the LIC classroom. The students will have twenty-four-hour access to the classroom in the Public Health building. They will climb the stairs past Birth Control, Vital Records, and Occupational Health to the third floor for a room of their own, and Adams pleads for them to keep it clean. She will join them for every Thursday afternoon class, but Kris Oatis, the administrative coordinator of the LIC, will be available to them anytime via text and in person four days per week. Oatis will always know the best way to track Adams down.

This class is the fifth LIC team, but the first with ten students. Each student is paired with an LIC student from a previous year, like Catherine Ard, whose interests mirror their own and who can, since they are on the other side of the clinical year, mentor. Each student will also be paired with a supervising physician in each clinic where they will regularly see patients. In the traditional clinical year, a student follows the patients a physician has already gathered onto her own service or into her practice. But the LIC works differently. Each student will build her own caseload of patients—based on who they see early on and who they seek out in their rounds. The student follows those patients for the full year, developing a sense of each patient's comprehensive health needs over the course of time. They will be in touch with patients directly, both to keep track of patients' care and to remind patients when an appointment is approaching. Their caseloads can rise to as many as fifty, but not all patients will be in the hospital at one time.

Adams runs through the basic information that the students need to know about the hospital's EHR system. The EHR needs no caffeine because it has no sleep-wake cycle. The students will check it before dawn, after sunset, and all points in between. She discusses how they will use the EHR to write formal notes and to stay informally in touch with each patient, sometimes by phone and sometimes by email. She discusses grading and testing, walking through how the LIC program will still need to keep up with standardized testing throughout the year. Adams sugarcoats nothing. "Med students have a reputation for not checking their email. You need to read your emails twice a day." Students nod and murmur assent. They don't flinch, but all the "to-dos" visibly weigh their shoulders down.

The room sits up straight when Adams turns to the crash course that students are about to begin. At the start of the LIC, students enter an eight-week, hospital-based immersion, an initiation into the rituals of medicine. This is like what their peers outside of the LIC are doing, but more concentrated—two weeks of internal medicine hospital wards instead of three months, four weeks of inpatient surgery (divided between general, trauma, and a surgical subspeciality) rather than two months, and a week each of obstetrics and gynecology—just enough so they can learn what a medical student does in a teaching hospital and how sick an ill person can be. After the hospital-based weeks, the students will settle into their repeating schedule of clinic and hospital encounters with the same patients wherever they receive care, before returning later in the year for additional immersions: two weeks on internal medicine wards and another week on psychiatry.

Maggie Kriz has questions. "I am still trying to get my head around immersions. I know we're just supposed to learn, but should I start studying for the first test now?" Maggie, like all the students, has been trained to think about exams and grades, the top priority of their past two years, as well as the four years of college before that.

Some of the students were birthed into this kind of vigilance about schooling, the transmitted awareness of the professional class that it takes good marks to earn meritocratic positions, but Maggie had to learn it. No one in her immediate family attended college, so she relies on the faculty to chart her own path. Maggie is from Steamboat Springs, a mountain town a few hours northwest of Denver, where it is more common for a native daughter to become a Winter Olympian than an all-season physician. Her parents—they named her Maggie Mae after the Rod Stewart hit—did not push her into medicine. She knew physicians in town—they treated her asthma, removed her brother's appendix—but they lived a different life than her family did. Like most kids, being an athlete seemed more possible. In Steamboat, that meant skiing. Maggie skied fast enough to make one of the town's competitive winter sports clubs, but short of Olympic-fast. Still, all the time on the mountain engendered a love of being outside. She started a high school environmental club. When the question of college came up, she applied to one university—the nearest—and enrolled at the University of Colorado Boulder, to study biology.

Maggie draws people to her with bright-colored clothes, hand-knitted scarves, and especially her open face, framed by bangs, and easy laughter. Maggie goes for earnest advocacy, so she tried politics after college. She disliked the cynical favor trading and quit to work at a homeless shelter. It was a wet shelter, where they accept intoxicated residents, and she saw people struggling with substance abuse, mental illness, and medical illness. They needed service and science from a people person, so Maggie went to medical school. She stayed in-state. She never wants to be far away from her family and her home mountain, where summers mean mountain biking and river rafting, and winters still mean skiing. Her current plan is to return to working with homeless people struggling with substance abuse, after she accrues more skills.

When Maggie asks about exams, Adams redirects her. She focuses on the immersion week itself, which aims to do more than prepare students for a test. "The goal is for you to get some foundational skills. How to admit a patient, to do an oral presentation, to write a history and physical. We teach you through internal medicine, because internists are sticklers for those things. The immersions lay the foundation for the rest of the year. So when you, say, show up on labor and delivery, you will know what to do. We'll do a ton of prep. We'll send out emails to your attendings and to the residents so they understand where you are at. Everyone will realize that you are LIC students, that you are different. By fall, when you come back, everyone will know that you can crush it." Then, Adams returns to the logistics of orientation.

There's still a lot to cover. She pulls out the next gift, individualized calendars, and explains each team member's training regimen.

During a brief break, the students compare their schedules. A student looks up from her schedule and declares, "I have a surgery sandwich! I start with trauma and end with general surgery." But they now realize that their two years of medical school have done little to educate them in the daily routines of a hospital. From behind her browline glasses, Sarah's eyes grow large as she says, "My mom asked me, 'What will you do all day in the hospital?' and I didn't know." The students nod agreement. They have made it this far and have no more knowledge than their mothers about what comes next. Maggie replies, "I'm excited for ophtho, but also a little afraid. It's like *Clockwork Orange*," and she mimes a forced opening of eyes from its aversive therapy scene.

Returning from break, Adams encourages students to look for patients to follow during their immersion week. They need to build cohorts with a diversity of backgrounds and conditions so they will qualify as physicians. "The best way for you to set yourself up for success early in the year is to cast a big net and look for any patient you meet during your immersion experience who will need continuity care and will receive it at Denver Health." The students nod but look a bit perplexed. How will they recruit patients on their own?

Adams knows that perplexed look. "You need to see these patients at least three times over the year. You will select patients, but it's hard to have someone to follow: a patient will miss appointments or will be at the doctor when you're out of town or at a lecture. But it can start from an immersion."

Adams tells about how past LIC students saw patients so many times that, even when a student graduates and moves away for residency, the patients will ask about them years later. Adams even knows of former students so committed to their patients that they will stay for residency or return as a faculty member. Adams dreams of continuity and deep knowledge. She asks the students to share the same dream.

Impressed, one of today's students leans in to ask Adams, "How do you ask patients to let you follow them?"

"Well, you can't ask, 'Can I follow you everywhere and stalk you?' But if you explain what it is, they'll be interested."

The students look at each other, sharing a flash of insight that a person must be pretty concerned about their health to allow a stranger into their life. Finally, a student asks, a little incredulous, "Do you just show up in the hospital when your patient is hospitalized?"

Adams reassures. "Yes, introduce yourself to the team. Students can add value by helping residents with transitions of care. Help them understand the patient."

The student presses further. "How do you build a cohort?"

"You need to look for everyone, everywhere. If you deliver a baby, follow the mother. She will probably need one visit. But, also, follow her baby, because that kid is a golden opportunity for follow-up. It's hard to build your pediatric cohort, so follow those babies." The students sit silently, as they realize that they will, in a fashion, build their own practice from within the practices of several faculty members. They will have to recruit patients to them.

"What do you do when your patient is on a service like cardiology?"

"Be flexible. Show up and learn. Help as you can."

Mackenzie Garcia interjects, "Do you need to email before you arrive?"

"It never hurts to email, but if your email is not returned, don't consider it a disincentive. When you show up, they'll be thrilled that you know about the patient."

By the end of the year, Adams promises, students will bring an intimate knowledge of their patients to each clinical setting. They will know what makes them sick, what makes them better, and why. Even more, they will know the names of their spouses, children, and grand-children. And, if everything goes as planned, the patients will know the students and their hopes as well. Being known will make the patients healthier and the students wiser. But Adams also warns them that medical intimacy needs boundaries. In the same hospital, a person can be a volunteer, a student, a resident, a faculty member, a retired volun-teer, a patient, a visitor, even a corpse. To keep the roles straight, the hospital provides many boundaries. The strains of being ill and caring for the ill can overwhelm poorly defended boundaries. A student can sicken herself by ignoring those boundaries.

More than anyone else in the hospital, physicians are permitted boundary crossings. To become physicians, the students will touch the bodies of strangers, set broken bones, ask after bodily functions that adults typically relegate to bathrooms and bedrooms, and—most inva-sive of all—see the patients outside the hospital. Visiting a few patients in their own homes is, Adams finds, the best way for students to really understand a person. A patient's home is the place where the textbook of the body and the textbook of the community meet.

"LIC students are in a unique situation," Adams advises. "You're going to follow patients, you're going to get to know their homes, their families, and their lives. It's such a privilege, which is why this is such a great opportunity. But it causes problems. We come from places of rela-tive privilege. You will be faced with opportunities to solve problems seemingly easily. To pay a dollar towards a copay or a bus token. And you need to think about it before it occurs."

For many of the students, dissecting a cadaver felt like the biggest boundary violation of becoming a physician. But they dissected cadav-ers in controlled settings. Visiting patients in their home tests further boundaries, because they will be in the patient's space, beyond the control of the hospital, where patients' needs for a dollar or a bus token will be pressingly real.

Adams registers the students' silent concern but presses on, distinguishing between being personally and professionally available. She tells the students they will follow the same duty hours as a resident physician, no more than twenty-four hours of continuous patient care duties and less than eighty hours of clinical work per week. They need to record every hour they are in clinical settings and check off every medical condition whose care they participate in. They will see patients with many conditions on many services, but Adams advises that internal medicine should be the foundation of their practice. "For surgery, someone has their gallbladder out, and then that will be it for the year. For OB, a woman delivers a baby and it's done. With internal medicine, if someone has CHF [congestive heart failure], you will see them again and again. Medicine is the easiest place to collect your patients. In your immersion, you'll learn how to admit a patient, present a patient, follow a patient on rounds. You'll learn what rounds are!"

One of the students asks, "Can you talk generally about the time to preround and when to talk to residents?" Adams responds, "Last year, they wanted students to be done with pre-rounding by 7 so you could attend hand-off rounds with the night team. Then you run around and meet the patients. At 8, you start rounding with your attending and then you round for hours and hours. Then it's noon conference. Afternoon is when you do the work. Then you go home and start all over the next day."

Adams reaches the end of what she thinks she can present today. She closes the orientation manual and opens a cardboard box full of uniforms. Adams passes out identical customized fleece jackets to each of the LIC students. The professional white cotton coats of old are better for ceremonies than daily use; the students don their customized polyester fleeces. They look almost ready to step onto the clinical stage. Then they are gifted the last piece of their costumes—a pager.

The students carry smartphones in their pockets, but the hospital is putting a dumb device on their waists. Messages travel only in a single direction—to the pager. When a pager receives a message—either a string of numbers or a few sentences—it vibrates or beeps in a manner distinct from every other alarm or text. The alert of a pager captures one's attention, and it sounds until a physician or student removes it from its plastic holster and acknowledges the message. It is a simple attention-extracting technology, calling for a student to attend to *this* instead of *that*, but none of the students can figure out how to turn them on. They look at the devices with the confusion attendant on a previous generation's technology and amusement at the perseverance of outmoded ways. Adams assures that, as amazing at it seems, pagers are still essential parts of a physician's costume. Still, she commiserates: "A patient once saw my pager and said, 'Doctor, even my drug dealer doesn't use a pager anymore.'"

Physicians still, barely, do, so Adams demonstrates how to check it, how to holster it, and how to clip it onto professional clothes and scrubs alike. Reminded, she takes a step back and tells them when to wear professional clothes and when to wear scrubs. When they wear scrubs, they must bring soiled scrubs to the hospital for washing. Sarah's attention is engaged by something truly useful. "Really? I could have someone help me with my laundry? Awesome." There are practical attractions to hospital costumes, to the doctor's life.

Before the group can depart, Dr. Kshama Jaiswal, a breast surgeon, rushes into the room and apologizes, "I was in the OR and the case ran long." With the Dansko clogs on her feet, multiple pagers clipped to the waistband of her green scrubs, and the oversized travel mug of coffee in her hand, she looks every bit a physician, even before you read her name embroidered on her long white coat.

Jaiswal is here to explain surgery at Denver Health, the action-packed specialty that the students will venture into first. The students will see general surgery, where procedures are elective and typically scheduled, and trauma surgery, where every surgery is acute and always unscheduled. The hospital is known for its excellence in trauma care and training. Many people still speak of the "Knife and Gun Club," the dramatic moniker the trauma team gave themselves. On their lapels, initiates wear metal pins shaped like a shield and emblazoned with the two eponymous weapons, pointed downward ominously toward the vital organs [9].

Jaiswal enumerates the varieties of trauma that students will see by naming objects of harm: guns and knives to be sure, but also cars, motorcycles, scooters, and bicycles. A trauma surgeon sees the world as stocked with deadly instruments. She underscores that the students are about to move out of costuming and into the real customs of the hospital. As a first step, they will need to be in the hospital for a 5:45 a.m. meeting. She keeps her counsel simple. "Eat when you can, sleep when you can, pee when you can."

A student asks, "Are there cases we should read about before we start trauma?"

"Trauma is like Christmas. It's full of presents you don't expect. It's hard to read in advance. Show up every day, but I guarantee you will see an appendectomy or a colectomy."

"Is your advice on trauma just to stay out of everyone's way?"

"No, you will figure out your role. After you see one, you will see how you can help."

A little nervously, another student chimes in: "How do you ask questions during a trauma?"

"It's a fine line. The team wants to teach, but sometimes they are busy saving a life."

A little more nervously: "I've never seen someone die before."

Jaiswal responds, plainly, "You will see someone die on surgery."

There's no other way to say it. And the students, who thought they were fully oriented, are now absorbing the weight of the gifts the faculty bore. The oath, the counsel, the uniform, the laundry service, the pager—all are full of presents you don't expect, the unspoken demands of the physician's life that you cannot appreciate until you fully become a physician. Jaiswal, meanwhile, looks to her wrist. She has a surgical clinic patient scheduled for 4:00 p.m. She collects her triple-sized travel mug, takes another slug of cooling coffee, says her goodbye, and steps out onto the floors.

It's not long before the students will follow. They have a few days left of practical training, and then they'll be alongside Jaiswal, joining her well-caffeinated fight to save lives.

Chapter 4

BLISS V. STONE

*T*HE STRUGGLE BEGAN with a fight on contested land.

During the 1858 gold rush, the land was home to indigenous communities—the Apache and Arapahoe, the Cheyenne and Comanche, the Ute—even as prospectors named it after distant leaders. At the confluence of two rivers, the prospectors named an encampment after the governor of the Kansas Territory: Denver. They named the expanse of mountain and prairie between Kansas and Utah after the father of their liberty: Jefferson Territory. Then they dueled over the divisions.

On March 7, 1860, two men, each armed with shotguns loaded with ball, stood thirty paces apart. The nation's Civil War was still a year off, but the two men were disputing over which side the territory should support. The judge of the local Miners' Court, Dr. J. S. Stone, supported the South. Stone shot first and missed. The territory's governor, Hon. F. W. Bliss, was an ardent abolitionist. Bliss shot second and struck the judge [10]. Bliss beat Stone.

Surgeons on the site did what they could, but Bliss's shot had passed through Stone's left thigh to penetrate his bladder. At the time, Denver had no government or school buildings. The prospectors had built the outpost's essential establishments first—bars, brothels.

To treat Stone, they had to build a new institution: City Hospital. When it was finally constructed, its ministrations included laudanum for pain, quinine for fever, and broth for hunger, but no way to put Stone back together. Seven months after the duel, Stone passed [11].

The hospital needed a morgue.

The hospital and its morgue endured, because prospectors kept shooting each other and getting sick, but its name changed. Moving around central Denver for decades, it has been known as Almshouse, Hotel for Invalids, County Hospital, Poor House, City Hospital, Denver General, and, for now, Denver Health. The place has been an asylum for the insane, a sanitarium for the infected, a health center for its neighbors, and a laboratory for researchers.

From the time of prospectors to today, the hospital has always been a place where rich or poor can receive care, and it has always been a schoolhouse. Today, Denver Health trains hundreds of medical students and a thousand resident physicians annually.

What those future physicians learn, and to what purpose, has become its own fight. Do you train physicians to patch up combatants and return them to battle? To study the sick and advance science with their findings? To reduce the social disparities that stunt health? To offer technical expertise or personal care? Medical students are asked to pick a side. Their answer would seem to depend on the available technology and the prevailing threats to our health. After all, the technology and the threat were drastically different in the era of *Bliss v. Stone*. And yet, even as medicine's problems have deepened, our fundamental answer remains unaltered. The gap between how we train future physicians and what our community needs is widening as we continue training doctors for the wrong era.

Today's medical school crystalized into its current form more than a century ago. In the late nineteenth century, medical education was—true to the era—the Wild West. The status quo was an unlettered apprenticeship, but reformers wanted to replace it with rigorous academic training. Across the continent, experiments flourished and faltered. In the forty years following *Bliss v. Stone*, five medical schools emerged along with the new state of Colorado, each fighting to advance its own standards and its own brand of physicians. Gross was a two-year trade school, named for an aristocratic Philadelphia surgeon, that trained private practitioners. Homeopathic embraced a faddish technique, teaching physicians to microdose poisons in hopes of strengthening a sufferer's immunity. Osteopathic proffered its own technique of manipulating muscle and bone, holding classes on a schedule so alternative they met only a few months of every year. Seminary, a three-year apprentice program affiliated with the state's divinity school, trained physicians as medical missionaries for public health efforts. And University, the smallest of them all, was built on a four-year curriculum centered on the research sciences.

The late nineteenth century was a period of experimentation about what it means to train a physician. Many medical school applicants could gain entrance without completing doctorates, bachelor's degrees, or even high school diplomas. Women and Black students, even in an era when both groups were profoundly deprived of rights, could apply to several schools dedicated to their education. If opportunities were many, quality was rare. Many institutions could not properly prepare physicians; others never tried, preferring outright quackery. The training was all over the map, and so was the resulting care.

Reformers fought for two generations to restructure medical education and practice. Instead of training future physicians in community-based apprenticeships, they would enroll them in university-based programs. Instead of welcoming large numbers of trainees, they would limit the supply of physicians. Instead of encouraging future physicians to develop character, they required excellence in research sciences. Instead of cobbling together funds, they gathered money from the era's monopolists: the country's richest man, William Henry Vanderbilt, endowed Columbia; the steel tycoon Oliver Hazard Payne similarly enriched Cornell; and the railroad baron Johns Hopkins catapulted his namesake university above them all. With the financing of industrialists, a handful of American medical schools rivaled the medical training at European research universities [12]. With the example of these elite universities as a lodestar, Progressive Era reformers gradually won over leading physicians, hospitals, medical schools, professional societies, and state licensing boards to advance a top-down mission to reform medical education. By 1907, the American Medical Association's Council on Medical Education published a report characterizing the quality of every medical school as either acceptable, doubtful, or unacceptable. The logic of the report was circular: only a university-based medical school could offer a curriculum based on scientific research in state-of-the-art laboratories, so only the university-based programs were acceptable. To operationalize the findings without upsetting their membership, the American Medical Association and the Carnegie Foundation recruited a man named Abraham Flexner to replicate the findings [13]. Flexner was an educational reformer, but no doctor. No matter. In 1908, Flexner was sent out to canvas the continent's medical schools. At some schools Flexner found decaying cadavers, at others it was the faculty who were decrepit, and Flexner called both out directly. When Flexner visited Gross Medical College in Denver, he wrote dismissively, "Its equipment consists of a chemical laboratory of the ordinary medical school type, a dissecting-room, containing a few subjects as dry as leather, a physiological laboratory with slight equipment, and the usual pathology and bacteriology laboratories. There is a total absence of scientific activity" [14, p. 197]. Flexner found the conditions at the school inadequate, and he recommended that it be closed. He wrote that even though several nearby states—Arizona, Idaho, New Mexico, Wyoming—had no medical school, there were simply too many medical schools in Colorado. "The state is overcrowded with doctors," Flexner wrote, so Gross should be closed (198). Flexner advised that Gross transfer the care of patients at City Hospital to University because the current situation was "plainly against the general interest of the community," an unexplained assessment that would alter medical training for a century (199). University was the only medical school in the state that approached Flexner's standards, so the City Hospital should educate only University students.

Spending less than three hours at some schools, Flexner nonetheless prepared a report that catalyzed a revolution in who got to be physicians and how they would be trained for the next century. Flexner was definitive in his diagnosis: only one in five existing medical schools was necessary. His prescription: admit medical students upon demonstrated success in the sciences as an undergraduate, train them in laboratory sciences at research universities, and expand their clinical training during and after medical school. His model for all of this was his alma mater, Johns Hopkins University, where Sir William Osler, the fabled father of modern medicine, had formed a rigorous training model. The medical school required a college degree and knowledge of several sciences (biology, chemistry, and physics) and languages (French, German, and Latin). After admission, a medical student at Hopkins spent two years intensely studying the basic sciences: the normal body in the first year, the diseased body in the second year. A Hopkins student spent two more years in clinical training at a teaching hospital, through serial apprenticeships to academic faculty rather than to a single community practitioner. After graduation, they lived in the hospital for a year or more of a post-graduate training program called, plainly, a residency.

It was a then-heroic amount of training that altered the landscape of medical education and practice by integrating medical training into the operations of hospitals. Third-year medical students saw specific patients under the tutelage of physician professors. Across the continent, medical schools were shuttered and hospitals acceded to research universities. A decade after his report, in 1920, only 85 of the 155 medical schools visited by Flexner remained in existence. Two decades after, in 1930, only 76 medical schools remained; in Colorado, only one, the University school, survived Flexner [15, pp. 243, 328]. The general interest of the community was best served by a research university.

Flexner settled the medical frontier so physicians could explore the body's then-unmarked territory. Germ theory was still a novel idea; the first viruses weren't discovered until the 1890s; a working theory of genes and DNA was still a half century off. For Flexner, this meant that the biggest improvements in care would come from increased research, increased rigor, and increased study of the body. So, on the first day of medical school? Meet your first patient: a cadaver in the dissection lab. Flexner called the cadaver lab the "essential" place to form medical students into the physicians the country needed, because it was the place "where the wise are brought to book" [14, p. 95]. Only in the cadaver lab could a future physician test his beliefs (and correct his convictions) about how the body worked (or faltered) with physical evidence. If there was one text that all medical students should master, it was the textbook of the body.

Flexner's fight to center medical education around cadavers created our health care system. Throughout the twentieth century, reforms advanced the efficacy of medical treatments. Basic sciences led to clinical medicines—antibiotics and antidepressants, vaccines and vitamins—that changed the expectations of patients and physicians about the clinical encounter. Many patients now believed that an acute illness could be cured with a short course of a physician's medication and an acute injury could be healed with a surgeon's blade. Many physicians believed they could *cure* illness. A physician could *fix* patients, twentieth-century medicine promised, if you followed doctor's orders. Life expectancy soared. Some people reached old age.

To take an example from psychiatry, one in four of the people admitted to psychiatric institutions during Flexner's era were admitted because of paresis, a crippling paralysis, often accompanied by grandiose delusions [16]. The cause was syphilis; the treatment was mercury. The adage was "One night with Venus, a lifetime with Mercury." Both divinities were ruinous to your health. Science succeeded where the gods failed. The *Treponema pallidum* bacterium was discovered in 1905. In 1908, a new treatment was discovered. Over the next decades, the treatments steadily improved until syphilis could be cured with a single injection of benzathine penicillin G. An intractable psychiatric illness became an imminently treatable infectious disease over the course of the twentieth century. Instead of a lifetime in an asylum, a sufferer could be healed in a single clinic visit [17]. It was all so successful that training models across the country, including Dr. Adams's, followed Flexner's model.

. . .

Catherine Ard followed only the first half of Flexner. Year one: anatomy, biochemistry, histology; year two: microbiology, pathology, pharmacology. But when it came time for her third clinical year, she enlisted in Adams's fight to change medicine. Catherine wanted to know how to repair an injured body but also where someone lived, what they ate, how they supported themselves, whom they could confide in, whom they worshiped, and how all of this affected their health. So she worked alongside Dr. Adams in her clinic. They followed patients together. Catherine found that they mapped the patients' problems—faltering organs, injured muscles—onto the textbook of the body, but she also sought understanding of how patients like Cecilia lived in their particular bodies in their particular communities.

"Cecilia's son had been shot in the head during gang violence activity. He lived but was now severely, severely, mentally disabled. Cecilia became his primary caretaker. She had also become the primary caretaker for her granddaughter when her granddaughter was four days old because her daughter had to go to jail. She had been kind of caring for her family, really struggling through all of this but trying to maintain strength and be a pillar for her family. Then she got diagnosed with metastatic colon cancer and had a total pelvic exenteration."

It's one of those medical terms about the body that belies the lived reality. When a surgeon performs an exenteration, she removes rectum, bladder, ovaria, and vagina in a radical attempt to save a person's life by removing every pelvic organ compromised by cancer. A body is rewritten by medicine. If Catherine were in the traditional clinical year, she would probably only see Cecilia in the controlled environment of an operating room, where all those parts were removed.

Since Catherine is in the LIC, she could follow patients like Cecilia over time, across any number of clinical sites, for a run-of-the-mill checkup, a first-time birth, a stomach-clenching cancer screening, or a last-ditch surgical procedure like exenteration. As she does so, a student like Catherine develops a full sense of patients' health needs, in an approach that departs from Flexner. For the past century, third-year students have rotated between medical specialties at rapid pace; every few weeks, they moved from surgery, to internal medicine, to OB-GYN, and so on, and they rarely saw the same patient twice. If a student is learning the body alone, the standard approach makes sense; it exposes students to more extreme cases and more extreme care. But the standard model also makes it harder to understand all those bodies as people—to get a better sense of what has brought each patient into the hospital, what their long-term needs are, and how physicians can best help. Catherine chose Adams's side in the future of medical education so she could follow Cecilia throughout the year in which Cecilia's body was revised by medicine.

"I got to know her well by following her through various appointments. We saw each other during some bad moments. She has a lot of problems with her ostomy bags after surgery and will come into the office just covered in feces. I got to see this incredibly complex social situation, through her experiences, these incredibly complex medical situations."

Catherine saw Cecilia in multiple settings and from multiple perspectives. It revealed to Catherine the multiple factors that had slowly eroded Cecilia's health over time. To improve her health, Catherine needed continuity over time. The LIC provided it. Now she wanted to spend the rest of her life as Cecilia's primary care physician.

"In getting to know her, it was like, 'Wow, I hope that I can continue to have these relationships and know this person for another 10–15 years.'" Adams wants that life for Catherine, but she knows how entrenched the system is, how our health system's players—from physicians to patients—are still working off the model in Flexner's report.

. . .

After Flexner's victory, the communities of physicians and patients, those who care and those who need care, diverged so profoundly that it created blind spots throughout the medical world. Patients and conditions went literally unseen by medicine. Medical schools became more rigorous, but also more expensive and time intensive. In turn, they became less accessible and inclusive. After Flexner's report, Black, female, and Jewish students only found admittance to early twentieth-century American medical schools during times of war, when white Protestant men were in short supply for the medical front lines. The pre-Flexner era proved to be a kind of high-water mark for inclusion: there were greater percentages of females, ethnic minorities, and middle-class students in late nineteenth-century American medical schools than would be found again until a century later, in the 1990s.

And the pre-Flexner-era percentage of medical students who are Black men remains, as yet, unsurpassed [18, 19, 20]. This was no accident; if Carnegie funded Flexner's report, the Rockefeller Foundation funded many of the reforms themselves, and between 1902 and 1919 it donated $1 to Black medical schools for every $123 it donated to other medical schools [21]. Women, minorities, and middle-class students were the collateral damage of Flexner's advance [12]. So were their patients; people like Cecilia are typically shunned by today's leading health systems. And yet, today's most pressing health problems are precisely those that tend to thrive in blind spots.

As medical science advanced over the twentieth century, many of the acute illnesses, infections, and injuries that killed people at the beginning of the century responded to treatment with predictable results by the century's end. But in their stead, physicians were left with the conditions that resisted simple, algorithmic care: the chronic illnesses and even more chronic health disparities that fill the problem lists of Dr. Adams's patients.

Adams seizes lists and manages hopes with okays to get through her clinical days, but she is befriending time to win a different future for medicine. More than a century ago, Flexner's victory led to a curriculum focused on acute ailments and isolated injuries, on knowing the human body from the inside out. Adams wants students to also know about how any number of social problems—from inadequate housing and employment to a lack of transportation, healthy food, or public safety—are sickening patients. Today, patients suffer from the endemic illnesses that sicken them, slowly, from the outside in: anxiety, depression, diabetes, heart disease, obesity, substance abuse, suicide. Unlike syphilis, they cannot be cured in one-off visits; they must be borne and bettered through long-term relationships that help people flourish, in care that understands where people come from, care that comes only with knowledge of both the body and the community.

Since the era of *Bliss v. Stone*, medical education has been about learning the textbook of the body. But our existing models teach students the body at the expense of the community. Today's students still patch up gun-shot victims, so they still need to know what bodily structures a bullet struck and how to repair the resulting damage. But students like Catherine also need to be taught to look beyond just the body. They need to reconsider, on something more than half-day visits, what Flexner called "the general interest of the community" for patients like Cecilia. They need to be able to draw on a second crucial body of knowledge: the textbook of the community.

Adams wants students like Catherine to learn two textbooks: body and community, together, through continuity over time. Adams is fighting her version of Flexner's fight because she knows that if you change today's medical students, you change tomorrow's physicians.

Chapter 5

DARK FORESTS

AS A CHILD, Mallory Myers was half-ready for the work. She had a physician's ambitious personality but a child's fear of blood. Her fear bested her ambitions.

Growing up in a Denver suburb with her younger sister, businessman father, and nurse practitioner mother, Mallory was a focused, dedicated child who admired her mother's work but not her mother's station in the health care hierarchy. "My mom is brilliant. But she doesn't like how patients don't treat her with as much respect as she deserves compared to the physicians. They say, 'Oh, I want to see the doctor. You don't know enough for me.'" When Mallory showed an aptitude for science, her mother told Mallory she knew enough to be a physician. "My mom said, 'You should consider going into medicine.' I laughed. I thought that was crazy. Then the more I thought about it, the more interested I got."

It helped that Mallory's pediatricians saw her through the travails of adolescence; she remembers them as "the best people I knew." She wondered if she, too, could help someone as a physician.

But the prospect of blood filled her with such fear that she considered engineering instead—another science-based profession with an ambivalent welcome to women, but without the harrowing intimacy with the faltering body. So she studied throughout middle school, never causing problems, never standing out. In high school, she resolved to be something more. "A switch flipped in my mind. I wanted to be the best student ever. I was very driven and I worked very hard." Once Mallory decided to be the best, she resolved to be a physician. "To me, the doctor was the pinnacle of being the best." Ambition bested fear.

College was premed at Baylor, a ring-by-spring place for many students, but Mallory sought her opportunities in schoolwork. Baylor, like many universities, provided premeds a clear map that would be comfortably familiar to Flexner in the way that it immersed a premed student in the research sciences so they could read the textbook of the body [13]. On Baylor's map, fall of freshman year was Biology I, Chemistry I, and Calculus I. Spring of freshman year was Biology II, Chemistry II, and Statistics. Sophomore year required Organic Chemistry I and Organic Chemistry II, along with advanced Biology, but they recommended introductory courses in psychology and sociology. Junior year was Physics I, Physics II, Biochemistry, and Advanced Biology. Along the way, there were laboratory sessions, research projects, volunteer experiences, and MCAT prep that ordered a young person's schooling. Mallory watched peers step off the premed path every semester, usually heading onto a less ordered path. The premed map was clear, but it was also designed to weed out the merely interested from the truly determined.

Mallory stayed the course and proved out, adding extra experiences along the way. She participated in bench research. She studied abroad in Maastricht. She read the prison literature of Boethius and met his Lady Philosophy. She wrote a senior thesis on the barriers immigrants experience when seeking medical care. She wrote about the benefits of having community members accompany immigrants navigating alien health care systems. Premed left her with an idealistic sense that a physician was "a leader not only in the health care team, but in the community. With that position, you have so much ability to impact people's lives—not only your own patients, but also the community you work in."

Mallory wanted to become the kind of physician who really knew her patients. What you could do in a medical encounter, Mallory saw, was about the mind and soul as much as the body. "There's the scientific part to it, and there's value in looking at the epidemiology and looking at prevalence of an illness to direct your care. But there's also looking at your patient as a person who has hopes and fears and trying to understand how that fits in with what they're dealing with physically. Because I don't think you can just look at one or the other. I think you have to put them together and acknowledge them."

When she received her acceptance notice from Colorado's medical school, she accepted immediately. "I was in a rush. I wanted to get in sooner and start that process sooner. I didn't really feel a need to go travel or do anything in a gap year. I was just excited to get started." Since Mallory's ambition bested her fears, there would be blood. She thought she was ready.

. . .

"This is the part where, from now on, you don't touch anything. You have integrity *now*. If you touch something after this, think of the patient, and scrub again. Do it for the patient's sake."

Dr. Stefka Fabbri is fluent in English, Russian, Spanish, and sterile technique. She knows how to get ready. So she is the one to teach Mallory and the other LIC students how to scrub, gown, and maintain integrity. The word usually means freedom from flaws. Fabbri means freedom from invisible infections that you can unknowingly transmit during a surgical procedure.

After another morning of orientation lectures, the students had conveyed their coffee-filled travel mugs across campus while wearing their scrubs—medicine is the only profession where you wear pajamas on the days you work the hardest—underneath their newly issued fleece jackets to meet Fabbri in labor and delivery. They have watched videos about perioperative skin antisepsis and sterile draping, preparing themselves for their first enactment in a year of enactments.

"Everything blue is sterile, so don't touch it," the first nurse instructs. The second nurse gives stage directions: anesthesiologists, pediatricians, and scrub techs sit on the periphery, while the med students stand around the patient with the obstetricians, under the OR's spotlight. The students look about the windowless operating room, finding no place to hide from the bright lights. Fabbri acknowledges, "It can get quite crammed." The students nod and scan the room again, wondering how not to touch the blue.

Fabbri greets the inexperienced students with the promise that they will take things slowly today so that they can follow fast rhythms tomorrow. The OR is still strange territory for the students. She directs them to hang their unstained jackets on hooks outside the OR. She opens a cabinet next to the hooks, revealing boxes of surgical garments. She pulls out caps for their heads and booties for their feet and then invites them through slab doors that swing open before her on motorized hinges. From the other side, a pair of nurses wearing worn-in scrubs and personalized scrub caps welcome the students.

Fabbri encourages the students to find a clear path. "It can get hot. If you feel like you will pass out, step to the side. Don't fall out on the patient." She shows them the sterile garments and reiterates, "Everything blue is sterile. If you drop it, let it fall."

Fabbri escorts them outside the room to wash basins. She shows how to activate the faucet by pushing their knees into the basin's belly. "You wet your hands. You brush your nails. You lather your arm to your elbow. Then you wash your fingers, your hands, your arms. Then you switch hands. It's kind of meditative. The whole thing takes five minutes. Top. Dorsal. Ventral. Okay. Done. Your arms are sterile. Now you walk like this."

Elbows bent, palms toward her face, Fabbri walks backward with a wide gait into the OR. She approaches the scrub tech at her table, like a queen to her lady in waiting, and begins gowning. As the scrub nurse silently performs her role, Fabbri explains her movements. "You walk straight into the gown she holds. Then she opens your gloves. You step into your gloves. The circulating nurse ties the back of your gown. You hand the scrub tech the card on the gown, turn around, and they tie you off. You are gowned. Now you can rest your hands."

Fabbri traces a square over her torso with her gowned arms. "The sterile field is here." Her body is a sterilized field; she has integrity. "The scrub techs watch everything. They will tell you if you have broken the sterile field. If so, step out of the case."

After the students complete their gowning ritual with the assistance of the nurses, they stand in a closed circle, comparing costumes to see if they are getting it right.

Sarah Bardwell asks, "Is my mask below my nose?"

"Yes," Mackenzie Garcia confirms. "Mine's not right either. I might have tied it wrong."

Fabbri adjusts their masks while instructing the group to tie wristwatches to the drawstrings of their scrub pants and to place jewelry in pockets. When the case is complete, they will undress in reverse order, reclaiming watch and jewelry last. They can remove the gown and the cap outside the operating room, but she warns, "We usually take the booties off in the OR because they get juicy."

A student grimaces and then asks about the smells. Fabbri admits they can be pungent but promises that a physician becomes accustomed to pungent smells and juicy fluids. The experience will help them become the kind of people who cut skin, divide muscle, excise organs.

Fabbri's eyes, the only uncovered part of her body, survey the gowned students for a moment. Their eyes are fixed on hers, and they look back silently, as the weight of what they are about to begin settles over them. "It's real. It's happening," she confirms. They will return that night to put their preparation into practice. Fabbri has done what she can to ensure that the students are ready, but each will walk into that unfamiliar territory alone.

. . .

The feeling of walking into a dark, disorienting forest is the stuff of children's fairy tales and adult's epic poetry. Dante begins the *Inferno*, "Midway on our life's journey, I found myself / In dark woods, the right road lost" [22, p. 5]. Many med students read those lines in undergrad and admire the poetry without grasping its midway feeling. The right road they are embarking on appears well lit, a round of entrance exams and prerequisite courses and admission essays with a clear goal: acceptance into medical school to validate all the premed work. Medical school initially seems just as straightforward, another four-year tour, like the four years of high school and the four years of college before it, to earn a degree. Follow the path through the dark woods and you will enter the Match with the assurance you will be a doctor on the other side. Unlike grad school in the humanities, with its convoluted paths with no guarantees of employment at its end, med school offers clear markers of success along the way to guaranteed employment. Med school is for those confident enough to run off into the woods by themselves, the kind who imagine journeys into dark forests as acts of self-discovery, if the way through is marked out clearly. And yet, as medical school continues, many of them get lost. Classmates drop out or are drummed out, become bitter or burned out.

After a discouraging experience is the best time to revisit Dante and his caution that dark forests, especially when the path seems straightforward, can turn you around until you are unsure which is the way through and why you ever wanted to pursue it in the first place. It always takes effort to forge the right path through the deep woods. Even then, you take on some of the forest's darkness and it clings to you.

Drs. Jaiswal and Fabbri both knew this. They were clear with the students: they would encounter death. There would be blood. There would be juicy fluids. But they also tried to light the way. Physicians and nurses would be there to help; and eventually, if they pressed on and did not sprint or flee, these students would be prepared for the work.

. . .

When Mallory started med school, she thought she was prepared. Med school felt like undergrad. She could do the work and do it well. She looked around for her ways to establish her future. She told a professor about her honors thesis. The professor put Mallory in touch with Dr. Adams, who was excited to work with Mallory on the care of immigrants. In those moments, medical school seemed as though it would be a continuation of her undergraduate years: laborious but rewarding. But medical school quickly sapped Mallory's idealism.

"The first week of pulmonology was just a lot of physics. 'Whoa, whoa, whoa, where did this come from?' I thought." For two or three weeks, she found herself disenchanted and discouraged. "I just did not care and I didn't want to study. And there was a lot going on at that time. School just didn't seem very important. I still tried my best to study, but I just did not care." Then the curriculum progressed through the organ systems of the body. When they arrived at nephrology, the kidneys interested her, and she found herself caring again. Less physics, more physiology. Medicine instead of engineering.

A few months later, she got run down again, during neuroscience. "It was the same thing. I just stopped caring. I think I'm really sensitive to people's moods around me, and if I can sense that everyone else is burned out, I start to feel burned out. I just can't help it."

Mallory excitedly entered med school with a sense of empathetic wonder, but she found her empathy working against her and her wonder snuffed out. During a seemingly endless series of lectures and exams about the parts of the body, she felt like she was being lectured at by the faculty rather than invited to learn. "When I talked to my classmates, I realized that those were also times when they got burned out. I think we were all kind of experiencing the same thing."

Lady Philosophy once advised Boethius, "Speak out, don't hide what troubles you. If you want a doctor's help, you must uncover your wound" [23, p. 8].

The first year of medical school uncovered Mallory's wound. She found herself burned out, but trapped in school by her own ambition. She could not take a year off, let alone quit. So she spoke out and, eventually, found ways to cope. She counted blessings. She cultivated wonder. She began dating a classmate, and it helped that he understood the rigors of medical training. She strove to improve herself. She pushed on through the dark woods. She found an unexpected reason to stay, as she liked her boyfriend enough to consider whether medical school could give her a spouse.

She needed a different path, one that taught her the skills to survive her calling while building the kind of relational skills good physicians need but medical schools don't always foster. She applied for the LIC with Adams because she believed that Adams would help her learn the skills of a physician who could stay in relationship with her patients and community, even as she fell in love.

. . .

In the afternoon, after learning how to scrub in from Dr. Fabbri, the students move on. They're taught to interpret the dark and light shadows of a chest X-ray. They spend hours practicing the suturing of wounds. These are skills they'll all need in the year to come, but not necessarily for the years to come. Only a few are interested in becoming surgeons and patching up bodies.

Despite his impish grin and self-effacing demeanor, Itzam Marin is so interested that he attended surgery rounds at Denver Health even before he enrolled in medical school. His interest is in a special type of surgery: ophthalmology.

Itzam's path started in Campeche, on the opposite side of the Yucatán Peninsula from the gilded Riviera Maya, where half of all the tourist revenue in Mexico is generated. Far less is produced on the other side, where Itzam grew up with his parents and younger brother, helping in the family coffee shop. Itzam loved home but left early to play his first professional football game as a fourteen-year-old. By the age of sixteen, he was playing center midfielder for his favorite team, Club Necaxa in Aguascalientes, and living in club housing. Every other week, they paid him 1,600 pesos. Every day, they taught him to wake early and practice in the morning and again in the afternoon. Discipline and teamwork were for the pitch, not the classroom. Even though Itzam was already interested in medicine, the club told him that football trumped schoolwork.

"I remember there would be tests that I didn't study at all, and then the grade would come back, and it would be B or A. I'd know that grade is not how it is. I'm pretty sure I didn't pass. But they wanted you to play, so they let it roll."

Itzam was ambitious too. He wanted to play in the first division, to play for the national team. But he saw that, even with continued effort, he would stall in Mexico's second division of football clubs. Necaxa, despite the wishes of its fan club *Sobredosis Albirroja* (the Red and White Overdose), was past its glory days; Itzam was merely a good player on a second-rate squad.

A friend told Itzam that second-rate in Mexico could earn you an American soccer scholarship. So Itzam sought a soccer scholarship.

Most players send highlight videos to college coaches. Itzam had no videos, but he had a family friend in the Denver suburbs. He stayed with the family friend for several months, took the SAT, and began looking at local colleges. He had the earned confidence of an athlete who knew the rigors of the professional game, the hard slide tackles that left bruises, the headers that gave headaches, and the hours of running that dehydrated, but each of those faded quickly into marks of experience. They were the kind of ailments that make you stronger, teaching you the limits to which you can push yourself. The soccer coach at a private university started talking to him about a scholarship, but when the coach saw Itzam's SAT score, college would have to be done somewhere else.

If Mallory took the fast road to med school, Itzam set out on the long path. Even in a country where one in six health care workers are immigrants, the route that each immigrant takes is often twisting, interrupted, or blocked altogether. There's the advertised version of the meritocracy, that the young can readily pull themselves out of poverty and into professional success. But Itzam saw the reality. One in five American physicians was born and trained abroad, but they are less likely to match in any specialty and, when they do, more likely to match in a less competitive specialty or in a less desirable location. Many excellent international physicians struggle to find a place in America if they did not train at a research university. Work is necessary but not always sufficient, opportunities are many but unequal, and you must start wherever you can.

Itzam enrolled at Metro State University, in downtown Denver, and caught up on college courses while practicing with the soccer team. Then CSU Pueblo, a state college 90 miles south and a world apart from the Colorado mountain towns for which the state is known, offered a full scholarship. Instead of soaring peaks, Pueblo is built atop a broad plane of lithified sedimentary rocks that gives the city a dry, high desert climate, more Albuquerque than Aspen. Itzam enrolled.

Even though a third of Pueblo's one hundred thousand citizens are Latino, Itzam encountered discouraging racism. The soccer team's coach forbade players from speaking to each other in Spanish. Two of the team's most talented players left the team, school, and country, returning home to Mexico. Itzam saw racism waste talent. He resolved that it would not waste his, even though he lacked the usual credentials demanded for med school aspirants. Itzam would find a way, through the discouragements, to follow his family dream.

Itzam's grandfather worked as a general surgeon in Mexico, operating in the hospital and running a small consultative practice out of his own home. When Itzam visited his grandfather, patients greeted him warmly and told of his grandfather's skill and generosity. The rooms smelled, unlike American hospitals, like the place and the people, because the community spilled into clinical spaces. Itzam remembers squeezing through tiny hospital hallways overflowing with sick patients while visiting his grandfather at work in a busy emergency room. He remembers his grandfather sometimes bartering for his payments and, when nothing could be bartered, often caring for people without pay. Despite the limited resources, his grandfather made even his sickest patients light up. He was there for them.

Itzam wanted to be there too. He enrolled in an outreach program that trains early-career students interested in community health, especially in rural settings, in the hope of diversifying and redistributing the health workforce. "It was a month-long intensive program. They provided housing and we had rigorous lectures throughout. It was amazing to meet people that were in the same boat as me, and colleagues that were always striving to be the best. People from that program made me believe in myself and fueled my desire to pursue medicine." Meeting people who shared his goals and whom he wanted to impress gave him the motivation to work harder in school. Just as with Club Necaxa, Itzam found himself improving as part of a team.

"When I came here, I had no idea how to study, let alone take tests like the SAT or the MCAT, or how to apply to medical school. Before coming to the United States, I never actually studied for a test or sat down in a library."

He worked hard but made friends as a resident assistant in his dorm and with classmates in lecture halls. One classmate, Andrea, stood out. He proposed; she accepted. He would pursue dual dreams—family and medicine—simultaneously. On a long journey, you need chance encounters.

On a visit back home, Itzam was helping at the family's coffee shop in Campeche when he served a visiting ophthalmologist. They struck up a chat. The ophthalmologist worked at Denver Health and invited Itzam to shadow him in its clinics. When Itzam arrived, he loved the surgeon, the place, and the work, a connection between home and away that made his dream seem real.

Now he is determined to take home with him. Itzam models himself after his grandfather, the man who, Itzam believes, possesses the secret to happiness as a physician: "a sense of purpose." Now when Itzam video-chats with his grandfather, he shows him the medical school's library, proof that Itzam has realized the family dream to study in such a well-supplied university. His grandfather would have liked to have subspecialized in cardiothoracic surgery. He wants Itzam to be a surgeon, even though a surgical match is more difficult. Itzam internalized the message. He wants to become an academic surgeon, the most prestigious kind, who is constantly being challenged by residents and students who are similarly driven. Itzam sees a bright path forward. He has already come far. He feels ready for the challenges he anticipates in the clinical year.

. . .

After the suturing workshop, Itzam follows a surgery resident down three flights of stairs, past the building where people wanting to enroll in Medicaid line up before its doors open, behind the engineering building whose smokestack is the oldest structure on campus, and along a curved concrete path to the main hospital. He arrives on the surgical floors. Tomorrow, he and the other students will start their immersion in surgery. The resident introduces Itzam to the team: acting interns, interns, residents, chiefs. Itzam will occupy the bottom rung of the team's ladder, just like when he started with Club Necaxa, arriving earliest and getting started first.

That evening, the students head back home, buzzing with new information that they'll have to act on tomorrow. Itzam returns home to his wife, Andrea. Mallory and the other students head back to their apartments. They try to relax, but all they can think of is the first day of surgery. The students wonder if the reality will live up to their dreams. They wonder if they can be authentically themselves even as they become physicians, if their path will sustain them through the dark woods, to the Match in the future specialty they desire. What Drs. Jaiswal and Fabbri were intimating was that for most physicians it's not a straight course into our deserved futures. The path alters mid-journey, looping forward and backward, while including everything that has occurred so far, leaving you on and off the trail during the same year. Ahead of them are forces that threaten to submerge them in the dark; they sleep, dreaming of ways through the darkness.

Chapter 6

LAYING FAVORITES

TO IMPROVE THEIR ODDS, students like Maggie Kriz beat the dawn.

"I would wake up at 3:30 or 4:00 for surgery. We had to be in to do numbers, looking at people's labs from the night before. I usually came in by 4:30 or 4:45 to do that and then we would round on our patients at 6:00. Rounding for surgery would take an hour. And then we would go into the operating room immediately from there."

"The OR is abrasive," she says. "You have a very real sense that you have someone's life in your hands. And it's hard to explain. You see it in movies and TV shows, and it's very different in real life." Doctors operate in scripted dramas, just like in real life, but rarely wait out delays for the operating room, plead for the anesthesiologist to prep the patient more quickly, or spend tedious minutes afterward documenting their efforts. But in real life, just like in scripted dramas, the surgeons were most themselves when operating. Those were the moments that mattered most to patients, when the tumors were removed or the ligaments repaired, and the moments when med students truly auditioned for the surgeon's role. If it all went well, Maggie would be answering questions and closing the incisions at the end, because the case was controlled.

Sometimes the case was uncontrolled. In one of her first cases, a surgeon found an unexpected bleed. "We were just going to do an exploratory laparotomy and take out the packing and sew him up. It turns out that this guy had a massive tear in his common iliac vein." The common iliac forms in the abdomen, around the fifth lumbar vertebra, and carries a significant volume of deoxygenated blood back to the heart. The surgeon recognized the tear quickly and applied pressure to prevent the patient from bleeding out.

"I just remember, he turned to me, calm, cool as a cucumber." The surgeon warned Maggie about how much blood she could see. "He was like, 'This is going to be a little different. If you feel lightheaded at all, I want you to go over there and sit down. Don't try to get through it. Don't sit on a chair. Sit on the floor and sit down,' which I really appreciated because I feel like he gave me this out that it's okay if this makes you uncomfortable." The patient bled and bled, as the surgeon promised, but also lived, as the surgeon hoped. The surgeon regained control. The patient lived.

You saw things, remarkable things, in surgery, Maggie said, and they were quite different from what was televised. In soap opera versions of surgery, the patient cases are brief and resolve at the end of every episode through the heroic acts of doctors. Those doctors live dramatic lives, in an and out of the hospital, but sudden deaths, endless call nights, and stairwell sex never muss the stars' careful coifs. Even more remarkably, the hair of soap opera patients stays composed as they develop conditions that diminish and disfigure real patients. In real operating rooms, the goal is to dial down drama, to routinize the surgeon's actions, so that they can focus on the drama of the patient's health. Real-life surgeons favored familiar routines over the dramatic surprises that propelled shows. Surgeons built playlists for different kinds of cases, insisted on particular instruments, and favored certain operating room staff. Maggie saw that the routines allowed surgeons to make literal life-and-death decisions as blood was being spilled, limbs were shortened, vessels were cauterized, and masses were removed. She watched as surgeons confidently excised parts of the body and tweezered them into stainless steel trays shaped liked kidney beans, leaving a little bit of the body, or sometimes most of a leg, to be taken out with the trash. "It was really interesting and eye-opening to get our first glimpse of all the different specialties," she says. "I had this idea of what I wanted to do when I came in. But when you're actually doing it, it's so different, and it's been interesting to be surprised by things that I like but didn't expect to like, or to have things that I don't like be things that I thought I would."

. . .

On the first morning of surgery, Maggie and the other students are all in the hospital by 4:30 a.m., carrying small notebooks so they can record details of cases to review later, and wearing scrubs on which they can scribble the urgent details in the moment. *K 125 O+ 4L Stat.* The students begin not with the patients lying in hospital beds but with the abstractions of the patients contained in Epic, the hospital EHR that is better at generating bills than adventures. Finding the patients assigned to the surgical team, they skim medical and social histories, imagining how to turn the patient's disparate experiences into orderly doctor's stories in the history, the physical, the progress notes. They want to know the patient in the way doctors know patients. The residents arrive and teach the students a way to defend from being overwhelmed by the work. The students can anticipate the day's work by writing an acronym next to each patient on their list that summarizes the necessary care activities for each patient: S-N-O-X.

See the patient. Check off the S.

Write a note about the patient. Strike out the N.

Place orders for the patient. Zero out the O.

Sign the patient out for cross-cover. X out the X.

The sun rises. Rounds, one of Osler's liturgies that endure in contemporary medicine, begin. A passel of physicians briefly visit their patients to review clinical progress. Students follow acting interns who follow actual interns who follow residents who follow fellows who follow the attending physician who assesses the health of the patients and the abilities of the team's laddered learners.

When they arrive at the door of a patient's hospital room, the attending physician stops before entering and gazes at a member of the team. The team member gives the patient's surgical story in two bullet points. Bullet 1: *Age. Gender. Post-op day. Procedure.* Bullet 2: *Pain. Meds. Appetite. Gas. Wound. Exam. Labs. Imaging. Plan.*

Forty-five seconds pass.

The team steps into the room, greets the patient, performs a focused exam, and discusses the plan with the patient.

Ninety seconds pass.

Check off the S. On to the next patient.

The students struggle to keep up, so they start feeling irrelevant on the rounds as the rest of the team keeps a breakneck pace. The team knows these patients. Students still must find their patients to follow and check up on, to add to their caseload for the year, so the students can become the ones who know. Maggie looks for, and eventually finds, one of her people on surgery.

. . .

That first morning, and every morning after, Sarah Bardwell could not find her people on surgery. Sarah experienced surgical rounds as too terse for knowing. "On surgery, they want you to say two lines. Anything more than that is total excess." Words slowed the surgeons' path through the wards, delaying entry to operating rooms. The words, Bardwell noted, must decrease, so the cutting could increase. The surgeons favored a maxim, *"Time is tissue,"* which indicated that you must move quickly before parts of the body died. Sarah intuited that the maxim reflected the ways they disciplined themselves. "People in surgery are brisk and brusque. They talk fast and you must listen fast. It's not cuddly and fuzzy in surgery." Sarah understood that the surgical residents were marshaling their attention for the patients. She perceived them as efficient, but thorough, with the patients. It was a different story when the residents dealt with students.

"Sometimes, I turned around and I lost everybody. I had to run around the hospital to try to find them." The surgeons spoke with her if she was next to them, but they would not go looking for her if she was not by their side. "It was run, catch up, listen, and ask questions, and maybe people will tell you what their reasoning is."

. . .

Before most people were even at work, rounds finished. Students joined surgical residents and an attending physician and headed for the OR. They positioned patients for surgery and then repeated the scrubbing, gowning, and gloving they had learned the day before.

The students were prepared for the cleaning, gowning, and gloving.

They found themselves unprepared for the surgeon's questions. The surgeons did not ask about the medical or social histories the students gleaned from the EHR. They did not ask about all the S-N-O-X chores. The surgeons assessed a student's clinical reasoning. It started simply, when the surgeons pointed gloved hands into the surgical field and asked questions: *What is this? Where is its blood supply? What vessels drain it? What nerves innervate it?* The surgeons asked about the patient's anatomy, or the procedure, or how likely a particular clinical outcome was. Inexperienced students were undefended. Smart students quickly learned defenses, like the 80/20 rule, guessing that the condition occurs 80 percent of the time if you believe it common and 20 percent of the time if you believe it rare, answers close enough to escape humiliation. Even smarter students learned to give the precisely right answer. If you gave a right answer, the surgeons ratcheted the questions further, until they reached the limit of a student's knowledge. Every time a surgeon found a limit, they told the students to look things up. The surgeons were teaching the students how to lay favorites, to play the clinical odds, because it could mean the critical difference between removing all of a cancerous tumor and leaving behind a vestige that can regrow.

While quizzing the students' minds, surgeons were also putting the students to work, extracting a physical toll on students and patients alike. Sarah Bardwell's first surgery was a transvaginal hysterectomy. "I think that my first thing that I took from it was how brutal we are," Sarah says. "Retracting in that procedure is just really intense. It is a brutal way to treat someone's vagina. Patients don't have any idea. You know, they wake up in pain. They know it's a surgery, they know it's dangerous, they know they have an incision. But the traumatic things that we do to people's bodies at surgery even in a laparoscopic procedure is . . ." She shakes her head. "That was quite astounding to me. It gave me definitely a new appreciation for people recovering from surgery."

"They're pulling, pulling with great force, you know? To do an open abdominal procedure and you are just retracting with metal on every part of this person's body, pushing all their organs out of the way. But it's the force that they do that with."

For the first time, Sarah is one of those forces, her body retracting for three hours at a time, while her mind is quizzed. When her mind gets the answers wrong, she thinks that her body hurts more. "My arm hurt so bad. My hand is going to fail. It's too bad I haven't been going to the gym."

After the patients' bodies are closed and the sterile fields evacuated, the students strip off operating gowns. After hours of exertion, they are as juicy as promised. They wash up, check off more S-N-O-X, and leave the hospital. They arrived before 4:30 a.m. They leave long after dark. They are becoming like vampires, purposefully moving about the world in its darkness.

At home, the students feel at a loss about how to absorb the day's invasive information. They realize how much they do not know. Instructors suggested books, even distributed digital copies, so they study bloodless books.

They return the next morning, rounding on their first post-op surgical patients. Then back to the OR. More questions they cannot answer. Book knowledge fails them again. The surgeons are asking questions that move beyond facts and into practical wisdom, knowing not just what can be done in a textbook but what should be done in the operating room. Finding themselves on the other side of this knowledge, the students receive it as a challenge. Within a few days, they abandon the books and find websites where they learn the information at pace, as well as treatment guidelines, drug databases, and clinical calculators they can access from smartphones between cases. They ask friends, nurses, and residents for advice. They learn clinical patterns and use those patterns to describe patients in the bulleted language that the surgeons speak.

Days add up to weeks, and they realize that they can take control of their encounters. They fire off questions before the attending surgeons can. The canny students ask questions to hide ignorance, to keep the surgeons from asking about what the students did not know. The wise students ask questions to engage, to learn, and to demonstrate that they can reason like a doctor. The students learn which questions to ask, which to answer, where to cut and when. They, too, learn how to lay the favorite, to gamble on the outcome most likely to win. Does the patient need a salpingo-oophorectomy or a salpingectomy? When? Which approach? Why?

They immerse themselves in the questions of each clinical service—four weeks in surgery asking when and where to cut, two in internal medicine weighing the evidence for which clinical tests to perform and which medicine to prescribe, two in obstetrics deciding when to deliver—to learn the basic answers of each service. Every future doctor needs to know when a person with abdominal pain should be admitted to medicine, surgery, or obstetrics—and each immersion is an education in a new way of asking and answering questions, in a new clinical culture.

They see that when individual physicians form groups, they accumulate a culture, each with its own axioms that teach what counts as practical wisdom in each clinical culture. A hospitalist at Denver Health collected many of them into a book, *Medical Axioms*. Reading through them, students find that internists are often conscientious neurotics who problem-solve to make the most likely diagnosis before it is obvious. *Better small than big.* Surgeons are often decisive extroverts who seek opportunities to operate. *Better alive than dead.* Obstetricians are often confident socializers fond of demanding work whose diagnostic bet is on timely delivery. *Better early than late.* As the physician Ernest W. Saward once quipped, "Every physician is a different kind of gambler" [24, p. 103]. As they enter the hospital each morning, the medical students imagine each kind of gamble and try out possible futures. They sense that selecting each kind of physician life bears risks—a surgeon risks being bled on, an internist risks being coughed on, a pediatrician risks spit-up, a psychiatrist risks being spat at, and obstetricians risk all the fluids—and each day it is time to try on each of those futures.

In the traditional clerkship, third-year students play at each future for a month or so at a time, trying out what it means to be an obstetrician one month and a pediatrician the next. It is just enough time to learn to dress like caricatures of the specialists: obstetricians layer blingy flare atop fitted green scrubs, pediatricians clip smiley cartoon animals to stethoscopes, and emergency physicians keep hand tools in their cargo pants.

During the LIC immersion, student experiences are concentrated, plunging into desired futures, so the costume changes are quick. Maggie, for example, begins with two weeks of gynecological surgery; then proceeds with two weeks of general surgery, one week of trauma surgery, and one week of ophthalmology; and finishes with two weeks on the internal medicine wards.

...

Maggie finds surgery as intense as advertised, but on the first morning she meets a patient she wants to know right from the start. Kenny is young, about Maggie's age, but he spends almost all his days in the kingdom of the ill. Kenny suffers from chronic osteomyelitis, an infection of the bone. A few years before, it got so bad that surgeons amputated his infected leg. Afterward, he traveled on his last leg, to the West Coast. That leg became infected too, so he turned back toward his midwestern home, to the physicians who already knew him. The pain escalated until he needed care in Denver, the most geographically isolated metropolis in the country, its sprawling suburbs surrounded by rural communities—some resort towns populated by the well-to-do visiting second homes, some agricultural towns populated by migrant farmers living in company apartments, each with limited medical facilities. It's the only major city for hundreds of miles in every direction, so Denver Health often cares for ill travelers who need care in transit.

"He ended up having to get off the bus in Denver because he was just in so much pain, and he was one of those patients who nobody really wanted to deal with," says Maggie. "He was in his twenties and was kind of abrasive." Maggie understood. "He's literally going through hell, something that is as bad as you could imagine. He had a wheelchair and had sores on his buttocks from the wheelchair, and his leg was severely deformed from the osteomyelitis."

Too deformed. In Denver, the leg smelled of cadaverine and putrescine, the colorless but foul-smelling molecules of dying flesh that make a person smell like rotting meat. The surgeons amputated his last leg, just below the knee. "So he's a double amputee. And also still actively using IV drugs. It was so hard to get him enough pain medication to where it would actually work."

But the first day on the wards, Maggie made it her mission to help. "I worked at a homeless shelter," she said. "I'm good with this population. I'm okay with awkward silences. So I just walked in there and said, 'Hello. I'm Maggie.'" At first, he had no interest. He didn't understand what she was doing there or why she was talking with him, especially when he was in pain. But Maggie was open: "You don't have to talk to me," she said. "I just feel if I were you and I were in your position, I would want someone to talk to. So if you want, I'm here. If you don't want, you can tell me to leave and I'll leave. It's up to you."

"It was funny, because he asked, 'Do you want to go into psychiatry or something? You sound like a shrink.' And I said, 'I don't know. I'm early in my year. I really haven't decided what I want to go into yet. But, you know, maybe.' And he was like, 'Okay. Well, I'm in a lot of pain right now and I just don't really feel like talking.' But then he said, 'But will you come back tomorrow?' That was my first sign."

Maggie returned the next day. One more day than a traditional student would have. It was only a start. She came back again, on the day after the next day. They traveled only a little farther together.

"And then on the third day, he really started to open up, and I think I was in his room for an hour or two talking about his life and how he became homeless because he's been homeless since he was 16 or 17."

Over the coming days, they talked about his drug use. They talked about his life. They talked about his tattoos. One tattoo quoted from one of Maggie's favorite childhood movies—*LEGENDS NEVER DIE*—a promise Maggie could not vouchsafe to the patient. Instead, she could promise she would return and listen.

. . .

Maggie selects the patients, like Kenny, whose stories resonate with her to join her longitudinal cohort of patients she will follow all year. She looks for willing patients with intense conditions that will result in multiple physician encounters. The traveler reminded her of the people she worked with in the homeless shelter. He reminded her of people in her own life who had died. She has friends with substance use disorders.

"For me, that part is personal. But I think more than that, it was realizing that there's this guy who's literally the same age as me, who had a similar life but went through a series of unfortunate events. I had so much empathy for him. You know, not every addict gets osteomyelitis and loses both of their legs. This is bad luck and this is society not taking care of things that we should be taking care of. I really connect with that."

Other LIC students find themselves selecting continuity patients in whom they are clinically and personally interested. Students want to conform to the culture of each specialty but be so authentic to themselves that they can bend the specialty back just a bit toward their own experience. Selecting the patients who resonate with the students is a way to be authentic. Students who immigrated to the country often take a special interest in immigrants and refugees. Students who lost family members to an illness often follow patients with similar conditions. Students want to hear about the paths these patients are walking and walk with them for a time, to see if they can improve those paths a bit.

The immersions also allow students like Maggie to see the same patient from the perspective of multiple specialties. She meets the patient who changes her life on surgery, but she will get to know Kenny on medicine as well. Interacting with the traveler over time, Maggie learns that connection and authenticity come through understanding, which is accelerated by the intense changes occurring in the hospital, the kind of place where you could be socially isolated while the physicians contemplate cutting off your last leg.

"When I first encountered him, it was just before he had his amputation, the day of his surgery. He was on contact precautions, which I think is another thing that makes people less likely to go into a room and spend real time. And so, we're all getting dressed up, and I'm putting on the gown and the gloves and everything and hearing his story. And then we walk in the room and he was lying in his bed, turned to the side, which now I'm sure it's because he had wounds on both buttocks. But he was turned aside, away from the door, looking towards the window, with the blinds shut. It was completely black in his room. He didn't have a TV on, didn't want to talk to us at all; really, it was very clear. We were trying to get enough pain meds for him because obviously he was going through an immense amount of pain, but he has such a high tolerance that we were trying to gauge roughly how much heroin he was using."

When Maggie and her resident walked in the door and began talking, Kenny said, "You dedicated your life to medicine, and now you got your doctorate in medicine. Me, I got my PhD in heroin. I spend my whole day trying to get heroin. I do as much as I can."

"That was the first interaction I had with him," Maggie said. "I think everyone else, they didn't explicitly say it, but I got the sense that they were sort of frustrated by his response. But for me, I thought, 'This dude is in so much pain. If I were in that much pain, I'd probably be that short and terse and abrasive as well, because he's just trying to get his needs met.'"

Maggie was too, by giving her life to medicine. She was working harder than she ever had, keeping vampire hours, but could already feel the LIC beginning to deliver on its promise. She was learning what most med students learn—the mechanics of examining, diagnosing, and treating a patient—but with the freedom to follow the patients who interested her. The one-legged traveler was not assigned to her by the team. Maggie personally assigned Kenny to her care so she could guide him through medicine's impersonal bureaucracies.

Maggie could see how the LIC would allow her to make a real difference. Over the coming months, she would see Kenny enough times, in enough settings, to know him, to advocate for him, and to think about how to become the kind of physician he needed.

"I think we did do good by him because he wanted so badly to get home. That was the journey that he was on, and that's where he wanted to be the whole time he was in the hospital. So I think in that sense, we did good by him."

Maggie already feels the pressures that the profession puts on doctors and how these pressures are passed on to patients. "I think the ways that we didn't do good by him are the ways that medicine doesn't provide time for residents to sit in a room and talk to someone. I like to think that when I'm a resident, I'll still do that, but then that means that you're staying until 8:00 p.m. to write notes. The ways in which we didn't do well are more indicative of the system than of the people working within the system. Because all the residents that I worked with had very good intentions. They just didn't have time."

Watching the residents, Maggie could see that in the next stage of clinical training the hospital would assign her so many patients, each with so many needs, that she would have time for little more than working through the constant tasks of hospital medicine. *S-N-O-X*. The residents told her to take time with patients now, while she has more time than responsibility. For now, Maggie has time to see someone along on his journey. She can feel time making her the physician she needs to become.

"I think I had this idea of who I was and which path I wanted my career to take. And spending time with people has made me realize that other things are more important to me than I necessarily thought that they would be, like talking to people and getting a sense of who they are to the core, not just what disease they have."

Maggie is looking at several paths in the Match. Kenny thought she would be a psychiatrist, but she suspects they will lead to internal medicine and caring for people with substance use disorders, caring for the kind of people she met at the homeless shelters and on the wards. Each potential path involves listening to patients like Kenny as they tell their stories.

"I like the intimacy of medicine. I like that you are interested in people's deepest, darkest secrets that they don't tell anyone, but they feel comfortable telling you. It's an honor and a privilege to be able to be that for someone."

Chapter 7

INSTRUCTIONAL CHALICE

*M*AGGIE KRIZ FELT the demands of being there for someone on labor and delivery. While the hospital often masked the power of clinical spaces with euphemisms—wards, units, rooms—labor and delivery was plainly named. Women labored, sometimes short and sometimes long, sometimes alone and sometimes with loved ones, to literally push another person into the world. Physicians delivered babies, sometimes catching, sometimes gently forcing, and sometimes aggressively pulling new life into the world.

It was on labor and delivery, her next immersive experience, that Maggie met Fatima. Fatima was pregnant with not one but two children nestled in the amniotic sac within her womb. Most women begin experiencing labor contractions well before the amniotic sac breaks, signaling the imminence of delivery. Fatima's amniotic sac broke before she began laboring. In fact, Fatima was at home when she suffered what doctors call a premature rupture of membranes. This put her twins at risk of a variety of harms, from impaired breathing, to dangerous infections, to death. Worse, her umbilical cord had fallen out of her womb, through her cervix, escalating the risks into a clinical emergency. Fatima needed to get to a hospital quickly, so she called for an ambulance.

"The ambulance called us on the way, and the resident in labor and delivery said, 'Bring her immediately to the OR.'"

When the ambulance arrived, Maggie saw something she had never seen.

"Her umbilical cord was hanging out and my resident was like, 'Feel the cord. Let's take her upstairs. This is crazy.' So we took her upstairs. There was a nurse pushing a baby's head back up and keeping her finger on the cord the whole time while we scrubbed in, and got ready to intubate her. It was just crazy. Fatima was alone."

Worse, neither Maggie nor anyone else on the team could speak Fatima's language.

. . .

Maggie shared the case of Fatima, the Arabic-speaking woman who hoped to soon be the mother of twins, at one of the students' weekly Thursday afternoon learning sessions. The sessions combined clinical concerns, like premature rupture of membranes, with communal needs, like how to care for a patient with whom you do not share a language, into case-based exercises that build their ability to clinically reason.

To get to the Thursday afternoon sessions, the students walk up the stairs to their home base on the Public Health building's third floor. The dusty space is crammed with hand-me-down supplies and re-purposed standing desks, each topped with workstations, telephones, and boxes of tissues. On a bulletin board, Kris Oatis has pinned the year's major assignments, alongside maps of the hospital and its neighborhood clinics. Next to a large blank whiteboard, Kris has hung a small framed and matted needlepoint sampler that looks like it was borrowed from the house of someone's grandmother, but when you read its rainbow-colored thread, it points to the future.

> There cannot be health
> without peace and social justice;
> and there cannot be peace and

social justice without
health.

—Vic Sidel

On the eastern wall, an oversized slab oak door opens into the room within an inch of the edge of a six-foot-tall black bookshelf, haphazardly filled with cram-books for last-minute studying, extra plastic spoons for quick meals, and powdered coffee for propping your eyes open. In the northeastern corner of the room, a desk is topped with a laser printer and another computer workstation, this one powering a computer display for faculty presentations. Next to the display is another whiteboard so the students can show their work, as well as, just like at grandmother's house, a collection of family photos, framed pictures of the first several LIC cohorts, and visual reminders to the current class that they can do the work.

They do the work together, in the center of the room, where students can push together and pull apart four tables based on the day's work. Around the table's periphery, there are office chairs for each student. Today, the tables and the students are together so they can eat lunch, catch up, and solve clinical cases in shifting teams of two or three students.

In the center of the table, a white plastic bucket filled with miniature candy bars sits alongside various textbooks, handouts, and one last grandmotherly object: a squat silvered bowl. They call the bowl their chalice. In the chalice's well are slips of paper on which each student's name is written; when a student's name is drawn, that student will answer a question from the faculty, solving the doctor's version of the detective's whodunit.

Today, the first faculty member is Dr. Vishnu Kulasekaran. Kulasekaran's jet-black wavy hair and thick goatee are still those of a young physician, but he speaks with the unflappability of an older physician, his resonant voice suggesting a depth of experience. He speaks only encouraging words, praising students when they answer correctly, asking them to reconsider when they answer in error. His kind eyes settle on each student in turn as he calls them together, asks for updates, and reminds them of office hours. Kulasekaran trained in North Philadelphia and now practices as a Denver Health internist.

Today, he teaches about the US Preventive Services Task Force's (USPSTF) guidelines, which aim to calibrate a physician's clinical judgment about when a medical test is advisable. Wait too long for a test, and it could be too late. Test too early or too widely, and you take time, money, and assurance from millions of people. The task force's findings are lengthy—like the dutiful students in this room, they always show their work—but are also summarized by letter grades. When the task force grades a medical intervention as an A or B, it is recommended. When they grade an intervention as a C, they neither recommend nor discourage it. Interventions assigned D grades are not recommended. The grades are often adopted by insurance agencies and health systems to determine which interventions will and will not be offered to a patient [25]. But most patients hear very different messages from the qualified and footnoted messages of the task force. They hear morning news versions. So Kulasekaran plays a video from a news show encouraging prostate cancer screening. The clip features lab-coated technicians and besuited and white-coated urologists saying that prostate cancer is the second leading cause of death for men, drawing blood from the cohosts, and then, off-screen, examining the host's prostate with a thirty-four-second digital rectal exam. The urologist promises that the test saves the lives of many men and encourages all men to get a PSA test when they reach the age of forty.

At the conclusion, Kulasekaran shows the USPSTF recommendations for prostate cancer screening. The task force grades PSA screening only as a C, and even then, only for men over the age of fifty-five, recommendations contradicted by the advice from the leading doctor on the morning news show [26].

A student responds, "Before third year, I wouldn't know what was wrong with this video. Now, I see what the problem is." Kulasekaran nods his approval. The student is learning that she cannot passively accept health messages; as a physician, she will actively evaluate health messages.

Maggie counters, "At least they were talking about public health and prostate cancer."

Kulasekaran nods again, agreeing that it was good for the news show to think about public health, but then asking her to consider the difference between having a urologist and a having a primary care physician make the case for screening. Urologists, like many specialty groups, favor their own interventions for each patient and often disagree with the USPSTF rating [27, 28].

Kulasekaran wants the students to think about the risks of testing—false positives, unnecessary procedures, costly specialty care—and how those risks multiply when spread over a population basis. So he presents a set of cases for the students to work through in small groups. The students read the case together, compare it to the USPSTF guidelines, make a recommendation, and then discuss it in the larger group. They get lectures sometimes, but most of their Thursday afternoons will be spent working through clinical cases together. They are not just academic exercises, Kulasekaran explains, because Denver Health keeps score about how well its physicians follow the USPSTF recommendations. Every day, when he logs on to the EHR, he can see a dashboard of his own scores in relationship to his peers. The dashboard measures adherence to guidelines, vaccination rates, and ability to control blood pressure and diabetes, as well as wait times and patient satisfaction scores. He can, in short, see how he stacks up every day. And, of course, so can his boss.

Adams has been silently thinking about how to bring the lesson home to students. The lesson is complicated because the science is contested and entangled in the complexities of American medicine, where a physician can find herself caught between recommendations and dashboards and the patients before her. Health care is a complex system, with multiple variables—the patient's health and history, the physician's talent and time, the insurer's resources and rules—which are competing against each other in dependent relationships. Learning to work in complex systems is the core skill to master in the transformation from medical student to doctor to physician.

Adams joins the conversation. "I always think that the scorecards are psychologically designed to motivate the doctors. When I see that I am even a couple of points below someone else on mammograms, it's like, 'Mammograms for everyone.'"

Adams makes it clear that the competitiveness of physicians, people selected for their ability to pass so many tests, will be used by the hospitals that employ them and the regulators who measure their care to change their behavior. Dashboards can become ways to weaponize a physician's drives against herself. The students nod again, but the lesson that students will have to mediate between the needs of patients, task forces, insurers, and health systems does not fully register this early in the year. Adams will keep trying. She takes the lead for the next lesson, selecting a student's name from the hollow interior of the chalice and calling on the selected student to pick the group's next case.

. . .

The chalice embodies a certain version of justice: opportunity and chance. Opportunity is whose name is in the bowl. Chance is whose name is randomly selected.

Random chance. Mere opportunity. These are the versions of justice that the students are being arrayed against. The needlepoint quote from Dr. Vic Sidel on the wall gives it away. While Sidel began his career like a good Oslerian, studying the body's red blood cells, he ended his career studying the community's social determinants of health. Sidel led the American Public Health Association, and his life's work was to study how social conditions affect health and to develop social movements that improve health. Sidel protested apartheid in South Africa and nuclear weapons in the United States. He studied the health of mothers in China and of teenagers in the Bronx. He lectured widely and often brought along a metronome, set to beat every second. Every beat, his obituarist observed, meant that "a child died or was permanently disabled by a preventable illness, while $25,000 was spent on weaponry." Sidel wrote books on how war, guns, terrorism, and social inequality eroded health and on how random chance and mere opportunity cost people their lives.

In one of those books, Sidel wrote that the philosophy underlying public health is social justice. "The goal of public health to minimize preventable death and disability is a dream of social justice" [29, p. 9]. Sidel wanted opportunities for health for all. He wanted opportunities distributed by need rather than chance. Sidel trained generations of physicians in the textbook-of-the-community approach, the study of the economic and social factors that affected health, including a Denver Health internist named Dr. Michelle Cleeves. It was Cleeves who stitched the final line of his *New York Times* obituary into needlepoint and placed it on a classroom wall as a lodestar for these learners [30]. The students receive the stitched reminder every Thursday and then must live its counsel every day in clinical spaces.

. . .

The next teacher to join their Thursday session is Dr. Julie Venci, a tall woman who wears her brown hair pulled tight into a ponytail that flicks back and forth as she moves quickly past the needlepoint on her way into the classroom. Venci directs the university's medicine-pediatrics residency, which is based at a Denver Health community health center southwest of the main hospital, and trains physicians in internal medicine and pediatrics. Today, Venci is introducing the students to community pediatrics: developmental screenings, dental screenings, literacy programs, food insecurity screenings—the early-childhood interventions that teach health-promoting habits whose benefits compound over the course of a lifetime. Venci teaches a two-textbook approach but assigns roles by chalice. As she begins, Venci asks the students to introduce themselves and the specialty they are considering.

Maggie says, "I thought I knew what I wanted to be: an ob-gyn. Then I did immersions. I really loved caring for IV drug users, so now I am thinking of some of these combined med/psych programs." Her first patients, Kenny and Fatima, have already set her on a new course.

Mackenzie Garcia reports an interest in family medicine, maybe psychiatry.

Sarah reports that she, too, is interested in family medicine, but yesterday it was her garden that interested her most. She planted eggplants, squash, and beets. "I've done it before. I have a pretty good system, but it took more time than I expected. I couldn't study afterwards."

Megan Kalata says, "I like women and children, not so much men, so maybe something with that. And for fun, I like to do yoga, bake, and be pen pals with my grandmother. Getting a letter is so much better than an email."

Mallory Myers says, "I'm not sure yet, maybe internal medicine. I feel like a different person after I work out, so that's important to me."

Several other students report an interest in primary care, either general internal medicine or family medicine. In this room, most say they want to join one of the specialties endorsed by the LIC's core faculty and by Sidel and the USPTF, disciplines that attend to both individual health and population health.

Not Itzam Marin. His laptop is open to the USPTSF scorecard and the developmental milestone assignments generated by public health experts, but he is also silently watching Mexico's performance in the World Cup. With his sly smile, he confesses to Venci that cheering for Mexico is what he is doing for fun these days. As for his future, he does not equivocate: "I will be an ophthalmologist."

· · ·

After Venci's hour of cases introducing various programs that straddle medicine and public health (e.g., Cavity Free at Three, Reach Out and Read), she rotates out.

The day's final speaker is Catherine Ard, the fourth-year medical student who has been seeing patients with Dr. Adams. She enters with a plastic tub of cut watermelon—Catherine always brings food—and each student scoops out a serving. Catherine talks about social determinants of health: the way factors like income, race, gender, and ability affect health. All of these likely influenced the care of patients like Fatima. Maggie wondered if an earlier community intervention, instead of an emergent hospital encounter, could have helped attain some of the peace and justice for which Sidel called. Catherine knows what the research shows: social determinants have more effect on a patient's health than a physician's clinical care. In one commonly endorsed model, clinical care accounts for only 20 percent of the length and quality of a person's life. Ten percent is explained by a person's physical environment, especially the quality of the air, housing, transit, and water in their community. Thirty percent is due to their own behaviors—especially alcohol and drug use, tobacco use, diet and exercise, and sexual activity. A full 40 percent results from social and economic factors—the safety of their community, their educational attainment, employment status, income, and support from family and friends [31]. A physician could, based on these numbers, make a bigger difference in a person's health by helping them flourish in the community rather than treating a specific disease that affected their body. It's Catherine's mission. She is here today to enlist the students.

Growing up, Catherine did not know physicians, and her own family avoided physicians because their care was so expensive. Even when her brother was struck on his unhelmeted head with a baseball bat, it was not enough of an injury to visit the hospital because, she says, "going to doctors was something that was kind of out of reach."

When Catherine did think about doctoring as a child, it was as an abstract aspiration beyond her parents' station. "I thought about it a little bit as a kid. But the response I always got was like, 'Oh, that's really expensive,' or 'Oh, that takes a lot of time.' And so I think those kinds of hesitations pushed me away from it for a little while." Her parents were caring but busy, having begun their family before they finished their own education. Catherine's father worked at a nuclear power plant, but he and his wife both went back to college while working full-time. Since she was the oldest of their five children, Catherine helped. "They were both working and going to school and really trying to make things a little bit better for us as a family. When we were young, things could be tough. You know, I learned the phrases of 'floating a check' to pay for groceries when I was a kid. I remember sneaking my siblings into like lunch lines at summer camps so that we could get food for when we were on summer break. My siblings and I really kind of became a strong unit."

She needed that sibling strength. When Catherine was bullied at school, she kept it from her parents. Instead, she used her parent's commitments to education to protect herself, asking her parents if the family could relocate to a more challenging school district. Her plan worked: halfway through high school, the whole family moved to the suburbs. The family stuck out more, but Catherine kept at it, until she stuck out enough to earn the support of her teachers. They saw her ability and encouraged her to realize her dreams. It was a long journey, but now she was realizing her dreams, helping to teach the next generation of medical students.

Catherine was in the LIC last year and found that the curriculum forms relationships with patients and faculty, but not as much with the community. Catherine tells the students she wants them to engage not in community service, an extracurricular activity in which a student delivers a benefit to the needy, but in service learning, an integrated experience in which students and community members encounter and engage each other. She hopes students will learn civic engagement, social responsibility, and interpersonal skills while coming to know people who are physically near but as culturally far from the hospital as Fatima.

"When you experience something, you understand it better, and it makes you better able to act. So we have designed two opportunities for you to understand and act," Catherine says. Catherine hands out several screening tools for social determinants of health and then pairs each student with a partner to evaluate a clinical case that is also a community case.

After her chalice exercise, Catherine introduces the students' year-long service learning projects. She assigns one group of students to the local Somali Bantu refugee community. Most of the Bantu refugees live in a long-neglected but recently gentrifying neighborhood located between the highway and the football stadium. Catherine assigns the second group to a local youth homeless shelter. She suggests that students assigned to the shelter might serve dinners, conduct educational courses, and engage with some of the long-stay kids. Both projects are textbook-of-the-community work. Learn a community, serve a community.

As she talks, Adams, like a proud parent, snaps a photo of Catherine teaching. Only a year ago, Catherine was sitting as a third-year student; now she is leading a course of her own. After Catherine finishes, Adams steps forward, saying, "This is a pilot. I'm committed to this project, but let us know how it works and we can change for next year." Behind her, Sidel's needlepointed words stand out in the sunlight filtering through the windows and onto a group of medical students pursuing the vision that animated Sidel's life—health, peace, and social justice.

. . .

Afterward, Maggie thought about how Fatima was doubly endangered; her twins needed to be delivered immediately to save their lives, but Fatima was also alone in a medical world that spoke a different language and confessed a different faith. Maggie dialed up a phone translator, and they did their best to explain what was happening. The message was urgent: "Your babies are going to be delivered. Right. Now. We need to take them *out*. It's going to be a C-section." But the woman kept saying, "I want to have them vaginally, I want to have them naturally." The obstetricians had to push back and say that it wasn't possible. "Are you okay with what we're about to do?" The woman said yes, but she also said, "I don't know what's happening really."

The scene was hectic for Maggie too. "It just felt so crazy," she says, shaking her head. "So we scrub in. The nurse is under the sterile towels, feeling the heartbeat and, as everything is happening, she's says, 'It's getting weaker, it's getting weaker, it's getting weaker.' The resident just has the scalpel right over the woman's belly, her big pregnant belly. And the nurse says, 'I can't feel her heartbeat anymore.'"

The nurse was at the foot of the bed, monitoring the unborn twins. An anesthesiologist was at the head of the bed, intubating the mother. Maggie and the OB resident were in the middle, over her gravid abdomen, waiting for their signal. "I feel like it was slow motion, but it must have been no time at all. Everything is going both very quick and very slow all at once."

Eventually, the anesthesiologist got her under, and "it was just, *cut, cut, tear, tear, tear,* getting to the first baby as fast as they could. The whole time that this was happening, there was no heartbeat through the umbilical cord." But then, they pulled the baby out, and it was alive. "It comes out screaming, just screaming."

A newborn's first scream, in any language, is the sound of hope. "It was just an amazing moment to me. A couple more minutes, maybe seconds, and that baby would have died." But, later, Maggie wondered about how coercive the encounter felt, how little choice the women had, and how alone the patient was. It felt unjust for her to receive care in such an alien environment, without anyone who could speak her language or practice her faith. Maggie, like her classmates, wants the screams of health and the peals of justice.

Chapter 8

LANGUAGE GAMES

*M*EGAN KALATA TEARS OPENS an oversized plastic sheath of gum, pulling out one silver-foiled piece after another, handing them around the table to classmates she barely knows. "You get some gum! You get some gum! You get some gum! Everybody gets some gum!" Quickly, wrappers are undone, jaws are moving, and joy is rising. Megan's gift cheers her new classmates for a late-afternoon hour of reading EKGs.

As the students chat excitedly about their experiences over the past week—the surgeries they scrubbed in on, the diagnoses they made, the babies they delivered—Dr. Jack Cunningham, a hospitalist, slips into the room. Silence falls as he passes out photocopies of classic EKGs.

Each electrocardiogram—alternately abbreviated as ECG or EKG (from the German *Elektrokardiographie*)—has a dozen line graph paper drawings that chart voltage over time. To most people, each drawing looks like random variations or, more poetically, topographical maps where placid plains are punctuated by pointy peaks. It takes a skilled interpreter to visualize peaks and plains as critical alterations in the heart's activity, and Cunningham teaches the skills.

Students know that an EKG records the amplitude of electrical impulses as they begin in the sinoatrial node and propagate through muscle cells in the right and left atria, the entrance chambers of the heart, to cause a forceful contraction that pumps blood into the right and left ventricles, the larger muscular chambers from which the heart propels blood throughout the body. Physicians like Cunningham measure the strength and timing of these impulses with six electrodes, embedded within disposable teardrop-shaped foam pads that conduct electricity when a gooey conducting gel is placed on the skin side, placed over a patient's ribs and four more electrodes placed on their extremities.

Learning to read the electrical activity between electrodes is complicated, so this is one of the eight sessions Cunningham teaches. Today, Cunningham teaches about the direction, or axis, of a heartbeat and the variables that can cause a heartbeat to deviate from its course. When a measured axis is deviated to the left or right, a patient's heart may have become dangerously enlarged on that side.

Cunningham encourages the students to work together through the EKGs he provided. The room's silence breaks. The students teach each other how to see the heart's impulses in the squiggles and tease each other when they misinterpret the squiggles. Cunningham stands at the east side of their table, waiting. With his height, black hair, dark glasses, and unassuming demeanor, he looks like Clark Kent, his formidable powers barely hidden by his costume, a white coat whose pockets are stuffed with papers, layered with a stethoscope around his neck. Cunningham is patient and deferential but also precise and exacting.

When the students look ready, he asks Megan to analyze the first EKG.

She answers systematically, calling out the rate, rhythm, and axis. She describes the P waves, which signify depolarization of the atria that fills with blood at the top of the heart; the P-R interval, which measures the time between depolarization of the atria and depolarization of the ventricles; the QRS complex, which measures the depolarization of the ventricles as they pump blood out of the heart; and the ST segment, which measures the interval between the depolarization of the ventricles and its eventual repolarization with the next heartbeat, which is indicated by the presence of T waves. Megan finishes with her interpretation: "an acute inferior ST elevation MI that has been going on for a few hours."

To be a physician, you must talk like one. A heartbeat is, to a physician like Cunningham, an electrical depolarization followed by a repolarization, which can be talked about in shorthand, P, P-R, QRS, ST, T—a cardiologist's version of the ABCs.

Cunningham is offering language lessons to Megan. When Megan interpreted the EKG, she followed an interpretative guide previously provided by Cunningham. She followed it well and, characteristically, with a smile that masks fear and determination alike.

. . .

Growing up, Megan was inseparable from her twin sister. They shared a room in their suburban Milwaukee home. They attended the same schools—a small Catholic elementary school, a large public high school—and were both accepted early decision to Northwestern. They were so much alike that Northwestern randomly assigned them to be roommates as first-year students. They pledged the same sorority and followed the same premed track.

Megan majored in biology but minored in psychology and global health. Her sister majored in biology and psychology—but no global health degree, the first on-paper difference between the sisters. But after Northwestern, the sisters both moved to Colorado. Their mother had relocated to Denver and returned to law school after a divorce, so her daughters followed. Both sisters pursued medicine, planning to be pediatricians. Med school started well, as school always had. Then it went sideways for Megan. She had planned to be in the LIC classroom the year before.

. . .

"You administer a substance and a reversible change occurs. Pain is blocked. Memory is erased. Consciousness is silenced." An anesthesiologist describes, in a confident combination of technical talk and medical koans, how to paralyze a patient so you can control an airway. The hair on his closely cropped head contrasts with the unruly strawberry-blonde beard that spills over the green scrubs straining over his generous abdomen. A camouflage-print US Army lanyard holds his ID badge down his back where it cannot impede the movement of his hands. In a single swift movement, the anesthesiologist reaches into the ceiling tile above the table, shifts a tile out of position, and hangs an aluminum hook. He quickly suspends a plastic bag of normal saline from the hook. The IV runs into Oscar, a C-battery-powered mannequin. With one hand, the anesthesiologist curves steel intubation blades against the base of Oscar's synthetic tongue so he can thread, with his other hand, a thin plastic tube into Oscar's ersatz larynx and, after securing the tube to a hand pump, inflate and deflate Oscar's artificial lungs. The entire procedure takes him seconds. Now the students try. The students fumble with their hands and their words. The anesthesiologist repositions their hands and corrects their language, teaching them the lifesaving physical and verbal rhythms of his specialty. Afterward, some of the more earnest students ask about the differences between paralyzing agents—*when do you prefer succinylcholine over rocuronium?*—while other students swap domestic formulae.

At the table, Maggie Kriz shares her kombucha recipe with Mackenzie Garcia. Mackenzie worries that she will blow up her home with the fermentation. Maggie reassures her that it is more of a digestive aid than a household explosive. Citing her mountain-girl credentials, Maggie enthuses, "I drink two gallons a day. I don't really drink alcohol, so when I come home at the end of the day, instead of a beer, I'll have kombucha."

On the other side of the table, Itzam Marin talks soccer with a classmate, happily alternating between English and Spanish, all while eating continuously from a Ziploc bag full of raw almonds and dark chocolates. He looks thinner than he did at the beginning of the year, no longer filling out his green scrubs.

In between these groupings, Megan Kalata sits alone. Among her classmates, Megan is always the student who seems to be smiling, whatever is happening around her. Her smile lights up her eyes, calling out for a similar brightness in the recipient. If that doesn't work, she'll try a joke or break out her secret weapon: she always has snacks at the ready. If snacks fail, she has even more ways to bring people close enough to her that they talk freely. Megan has one of the best skills a physician can have—the ability to win the confidences of people from all walks of life—but it is a skill rewarded more in medical practice than in medical school.

. . .

Megan faltered at the most rewarded skill of med school: testing. Megan was accepted into last year's LIC and then took the first of three big tests from the United States Medical Licensing Exam. The standardized exam called Step 1 consists of hundreds of multiple-choice questions that are taken in three separate daylong sessions at different stages of a future physician's training. Students usually take Step 1 before entering their clinical year, Step 2 before medical school graduation, and Step 3 before completing residency. The first step is the most critical, even though it is the worst measure. Step 3 assesses the skills of a physician and correlates with clinical ability. Step 1 gatekeeps students and correlates with scientific knowledge and test-taking skills. While there are more effective ways to predict the success of a medical student as a practicing physician—verbal ability, humanistic concern, and performance in the clinical year—Step 1 is the most efficient way to stratify a med student in relationship to other applicants and the current members of the specialty to which she is attempting to match [13]. Since the salary differential between the least and most competitive specialties can be fivefold, fortunes are at stake.

Students have gotten the message—outscore the mean to secure your future. One in twenty medical students fails the exam outright. Even more medical students experience anxiety over the prospect of the exam. A growing number of students, sometimes a quarter of the class at the University of Colorado, delay entry into the clinical years to extend study time for Step 1.

Megan never wanted a delay, but when she unwrapped her test report, it read FAIL in block letters, like a stop sign at an educational intersection. It added an *if* to her dream. She searched for the reasons why, but they all felt like the post hoc explanations and face-saving justifications proffered after the end of a relationship. You need a story to explain how the relationship you thought was *the one* became *the last one*.

You make up a story, but it's the feeling of failure that remains real. Being a good student is how most medical students identified themselves in the world. They could be picked last for playground teams in elementary school, passed over for party invitations in middle school, or rejected by high school crushes, just as long as they excelled in the classroom in every grade. In the classroom, the pride a future med student takes in translating effort into test scores becomes an identity. Through the striving and the scoring and the sorting, they are being groomed for the meritocracy, where identity is contingent on performance.

So failing Step 1, a demerit from the meritocracy, feels like a sin against your station. And when you are training for a caring profession, a FAIL makes you feel neither caring enough nor smart enough to stay. When a student fails, they often worry that the med school wasted its efforts on them. Failing the step, a student's sleep is often fractured and their mood fretful. Night and day, anxious concerns intrude upon a student's thoughts. *What was the difference between CD2 and CD28 on T lymphocytes? Who named these? Why cannot I remember? Why I am so bad at this? Who am I if I fail again?* The answer to the last one seems apparent: a second FAIL notice will certify a student as a failure, as an ex-med student. The reassuring joke of medical school—Q: *What do you call a medical student who finishes at the bottom of their class?* A: *Doctor*—has no reassurance for those whose failure places them below the bottom. If you fail out of medical school, there is not much to be done with a partial medical school education, except pay off student loans for the remainder of your days.

. . .

Living as a physician with an *if* can be done. Patients never ask about Step 1 scores, only if you can and will care for them. If you work hard for patients, you can learn the language of a physician. Speak it well enough to pass the exam, and you can enter the clinical year. Work hard and well in the clinical year, and you are eligible for the Match and your future.

Learning to talk like a physician is the only way to realize medical dreams. By some estimates, students learn fifty-five thousand new words in medical school [32]. The sheer volume of words in medicine's complex language game is an invitation for a student to regress. They have all reached adulthood, but the average American has a vocabulary of only twenty-five thousand to thirty-five thousand words. Medical students enter a new society with so many new words that it can make them feel like children in the company of adults speaking a made-up language to keep them out of the conversation. *Pick a part of the body. Make up a bunch of acronyms. Add -ology to the end of everything. Talk about doctor this, nurse this, resident that.* Medical language makes children out of adults by taking students like Megan and speaking to them in a new language. Most students stumble along the way but learn the language. A heartbeat becomes an electrical impulse causing a depolarization followed by a repolarization. A memory is erased by propofol because it induces hyporesponsiveness of the hippocampus. As they learn the languages, students try out roles to belong. A medical student becomes a doctor who becomes an obstetrician or ophthalmologist. A medical student learns to speak the language, so she can find her way through the curious worlds of medicine.

It is hard to find your way alone, so teachers like Cunningham use teamwork to teach the students medical language and to give them company as they work toward a common goal. Thursday afternoon sessions provide public opportunities to master the medical language with each other before they speak doctor on the wards and in the clinics. In between classes, they share textbooks that teach the language and answer practice questions that reinforce the language. Then they play the game itself, encountering patients in a variety of clinical environments.

Megan's Monday began with rounds with both the internal medicine and surgery teams in the main hospital, followed by an afternoon in a pediatrics clinic. Tuesday morning started with a two-hour quality improvement conference, followed by a cross-town commute to a family medicine clinic for prenatal visits, then back across town for an afternoon psychiatry clinic. Wednesday brought predawn meetings with the surgeons, then a day on the psychiatric emergency service. On Thursday morning, she was in an outlying clinic with an obstetrician, before afternoon chalice exercises until 4:30 p.m., after which she will return to the hospital for more internal medicine rounds. On it goes—and that is just her daytime schedule—and at each encounter, she learns to talk like a physician, a year late, but in her time.

. . .

For some students who fail Step 1, there was a warning sign along the way—a course failure, a mental illness, a personal crisis—and other times it is, as it was for Megan, an isolated failure occurring years (and tens of thousands of dollars of student loans) along the way toward a successful career. The failure wounded Megan. It even took her off cycle from her twin sister, who continued to pediatrics.

Alone, Megan found that her dream remained. She took a leave of absence from the medical school. She gathered herself around her dream and added new elements to it.

The university's public health school offered a one-year master's degree, so she spent her days earning a master's in public health, working on a community-based infant mortality research project. She quantified racial disparities. She visited homeless shelters and needle exchange programs. She studied policymaking and lobbying.

Megan enjoyed it, but still wants to do so as a physician because she loves how a medical encounter is an "intimate relationship that people can have." She marvels at the amount of trust people give to physicians and what it induces in a physician, saying that she needs "to be constantly learning and curious" to deserve and maintain that trust. So she spent her nights relearning the material on Step 1. *Krebs cycle. Brachial plexus. Virchow's triad.* She needed to pass to return to clinical year, to resume her interrupted dream.

Before medical school, the dream was pediatrics. She wanted to keep kids safe and give them a healthy start. The year away shifted her dream. She volunteered as a doula, accompanying women across the hospital, from infertility clinics to prenatal visits to birthing rooms, and felt the advantage of following women over time. She would enter the room, pull up a chair, introduce herself to everyone in the room, and ask how she could help. There were a few things that helped most people, so she would try those first while building enough trust to tailor her suggestions to the laboring mother. If she built trust with a woman during early labor, the woman would look around the room for her when it came time to deliver, even though the room was now filled with more experienced clinicians. The experience left Megan dreaming of being one of the clinicians. She loves labor because of "the relationship that you build with patients, the kind of different experiences that you have with them that you can be there during one of the most exciting and special moments of their lives and you can also be there with them when really hard things are happening too." She realized, "I could help women but also be helping their future children." She built on clinical experiences with her public health training. She learned community research techniques and how to lead change. "I'm genuine about this and I'm passionate and I want to be here and to understand and to learn from these women and hear what they have to say." She assembled every experience she needs to be an obstetrician—except one.

Her new dream is qualified by that *if.* Step 1 is the only nationwide examination most students complete before applying to residencies. Residencies are overwhelmed by aspirants, often receiving a hundred applications for each position, so they need a simple measure to decide whom to consider. Many residencies settle on Step 1 scores to sort students into the medical hierarchy. Competitive residencies like OB/GYN, especially the most prestigious, are loath to risk even an interview on an applicant who scores below the mean on Step 1 or Step 2. Many residencies will never even read the application of a student who received a FAIL. Megan may have to settle for a residency where deliveries are less common, like family medicine, or risk going without any residency. Without a residency, a student's efforts lead to, at best, an unplanned career and, at worst, debilitating debt that can never be repaid because they are unable to practice as a physician without completing at least some residency training. Over the past two decades, the number of American medical students has increased by over 50 percent, but the number of residency spots has only grown by 1 percent annually, so there is a gap between the number of students who complete medical school as doctors and those who will be able to train as physicians. About nineteen in twenty American MD students match, about nine in ten American DO students match, and two in three international medical graduates match [33, 34].

To secure her Match, Megan has taken an extra year, but it was a year well spent in public health and as a doula. She has made it to her clinical year and axis deviation and succinylcholine versus rocuronium and all the other language lessons the faculty are offering. She will not graduate with her original class, but she is resolved to graduate with the students with whom she is sharing gum. The other students, still on schedule, are assured of matching into some specialty. Megan does not feel the same assurance. She is not guaranteed a future as a physician. No matter. Megan is determined to match, no matter how long it takes. She will be a physician.

Chapter 9

DAY-TIGHT
COMPARTMENTS

*M*ALLORY MYERS IS FAST but confides that her fast is not Dr. Adams fast. "I always worry that I am being too slow." Mallory usually sees three patients in each half-day clinic, a fraction of the number Adams sees. Adams supervises Mallory for internal medicine, usually Mondays at Westside, Tuesdays in the HIV clinic. Adams is currently blazing through another patient alone, while Mallory sits in the bullpen preparing herself for the next patient. She logs on to the EHR and begins prepping a clinic note. Ten seconds of precision typing. Ten seconds of pointing and clicking with the mouse. Ten seconds of precision typing. Ten seconds of pointing and clicking with the mouse. Adams returns to the workroom and interrupts.

"Let's do feedback now, otherwise I will forget. You did a good job, but here are a few things. I know we need to manage time, but if a patient brings in only three things, we can cover them all. You asked about diet and exercise, but I've learned to ask, 'What is the one thing you would like to change about the way you eat?' Does that make sense?"

"That is helpful. She was a little grumpy."

"She is always a little grumpy. Her daughter is in prison. Her grandchildren are in the custody of a friend. But the friend is working constantly, so she is raising her grandchildren. I'd say she is appropriately grumpy."

Mallory nods at Adams's reminder that they need to understand a patient's life to understand her behavior.

To meet a patient so well that you understand why she is grumpy, a medical student needs a mentor who teaches a student how a patient's body and community relate, while guiding the student to the specialty that will become her life's practice, organizing her days and nights into concentrated doses of encountering the ill. Adams will be her teacher along the way, following the most famous of all physician teachers. Sir William Osler, the Johns Hopkins physician who was the first to train medical students at the bedside, counseled students that "the way of life that I preach is a habit to be acquired gradually by long and steady repetition. It is the practice of living for the day only, and for the day's work, *Life in day-tight compartments*" [35, pp. 13–14]. The third year is when a student picks the day-tight compartment she will pursue in the Match.

Adams was born to lead students into medicine's compartments. She has several uncles and a cousin who are physicians. Her only sibling is a family physician. Adams is a fourth-generation physician, albeit the first woman in the line, trained on the textbook of the body.

She models herself after her father, an internist like Osler, for whom medicine was a one-on-one activity of serving patients over a lifetime. His own father had been a Congregationalist United Church of Christ minister, and they moved often for different church assignments, relocating where they were needed. Her father was raised to serve but found a way to do so without living in church housing. As a college senior, he joined a civil rights march, from Selma to Montgomery, and then went on to medical school in Iowa City, where the future Dr. Jim Adams met the future Mrs. Adams, a social worker. He was conscripted, but in lieu of Vietnam, they served a medical deployment that moved them around as much as a circuit-riding minister: two years at a public service hospital on Staten Island, a year on a Navajo reservation in Gallup, and two years in Sacramento to complete his internal medicine training. Adams's parents were following another bit of Oslerian advice: "The all-important matter is to get breadth of view as early as possible, and this is difficult without travel" [36, p. 142]. Osler added to this advice his own teacher's aphoristic advice about working hard when you are young to reap the rewards when established, saying that an internist should strive ten years for bread, strive ten years for bread and butter, and then dine for twenty years on cakes and ale [37]. For Adams's parents, their years riding the medical circuit, accumulating the diverse experiences that make an internist, were the bread years.

Afterward, they were ready to settle down, so he began his butter years at a Kaiser practice in a southwest Denver suburb and his wife birthed Adams. She cannot recall becoming aware that her father was a physician. Being a physician was "so ingrained. It was what we talked about. It was what he did. It was just always there. . . . If you asked him to describe himself, 'physician' would be one of the first words out of his mouth."

While many physicians from her father's generation, now safely in their cake and ale years, are bitter over the changes in medical practice, Adams says her father's love of medicine never soured. He was sustained by his love of patients, spending a half century as their physician in the same office, with the same staff. It was service, but in a scientific, rationalized way. And so he raised their two children in their own home instead of a church parsonage; weekends meant skiing instead of Sunday School. Weekdays were for medicine, practiced within a larger network in which he could refer patients for the specialty services they needed.

While Adams grew up admiring her father, she only realized she wanted to be a physician in college. "I knew I was interested in medicine, but my idea of medicine largely came from what I had seen my dad do." It was junior year, semester abroad in Kenya, that changed her vision of medicine and her future. She saw how medicine could be a pursuit of justice. She had a direction. She would be a physician who addressed the inequity of the world. She returned from Kenya determined. "I came back and really wanted to make a difference in the world." After graduation, she came home, spent a year in AmeriCorps, and took the MCAT. She took it again. She was accepted at her state medical school, the University of Colorado School of Medicine.

She enrolled. The curriculum was "the old, old curriculum," the one that would have been familiar to all three generations before her and to old Osler himself. On the first day of med school, she was assigned alphabetically into a group of six classmates—all of their last names began with A or B—to dissect an elderly woman's corpse. Her first patient was deceased, her first textbook a corpse in a dissecting room. But despite that very direct bodily contact with sickness and death, her memories of the preclinical years are mostly from the library, hours spent studying the lessons her cadaver taught, with classmates who became friends. She lived each day in Osler's day-tight compartments: library, laboratory, lecture hall. It was more work than college, but Adams found it fun.

What captured the parts of her heart awakened by Kenya were the people she met in third year, the year when medical students must give up their neat compartments in exchange for some of the messiness of medical practice. Adams embarked on the medical student version of circuit riding, spending half of her three-month internal medicine clerkship 200 miles south of the medical school, in Alamosa, a town of fewer than ten thousand souls along the Rio Grande in the San Luis Valley, the highest and largest agricultural valley in the world. Then, she spent her monthlong family medicine clerkship up north near the Wyoming border, in Craig, where the fields are fracked instead of farmed and the locals declare the place the elk-hunting capital of the world.

In Craig, Adams lived the life of a rural physician, sharing his work and his house. "We'd deliver babies together in the middle of the night. I did an appendectomy with him, and I lived in his basement so he would just knock on my door and be like, 'Come on, we're going to the hospital.' He loved to duck hunt. On the weekends he would take me out." She had never held a gun before. Now she watched as her supervising physician hunted with his shotgun. "He had this very strong feeling that if you killed an animal, you had to eat it. He would take the ducks and put them in a crockpot on Sunday night and pour fruit cocktail over them, and then let it simmer all day on Monday. And then it would just be this like sludge of grease and disgusting mess and even he had to choke it down. We'd sit there and eat it all week and then go duck hunting again the next weekend." Adams fondly recalls all she learned as a medical student living in the borrowed basement room of a bachelor physician's home, eating duck cooked in fruit cocktail, and getting up in the middle of the night to deliver babies.

Wanting that kind of community, minus the duck fat, she spent the remainder of her third year at Denver Health. "I just loved Denver Health. I loved the patients, I loved the people, I loved the vibe of it and I requested it for all my subsequent rotations."

It helped to root herself in a place. The next step was to sort out her future specialty. She disliked the operating room; she struck surgery off the list. She disliked making children cry during her examination; she omitted pediatrics. She disliked the difficulty of trying to connect with the mentally ill; she nixed psychiatry. She liked forming relationships with her patients; she settled on becoming a primary care physician. She wanted to form relationships over time, to bend the arc of a person's life toward health. The joy her father found in primary care had sustained him; now it would sustain her.

Adams was initially reluctant to select internal medicine because it was her father's specialty. "The teenager in me sort of wanted to be my own person. I kind of wanted to branch out on my own and do something different." A strong candidate, she received residency interviews all over the country. On the interview trail, she says, her choice became "very clear." When she visited internal medicine programs, she was "super excited," and when she visited family medicine programs, she felt to herself, "these aren't my people." In the Match, she selected internal medicine for her compartment. "I think so much of your career choice is who you connect with, and who ends up being a great mentor and role model for you. For me, those were internists." Today, she tells her medical students that you know you have found your future specialty when you have found the people with whom you can be in a compartment.

She found her mentors at the University of California, San Francisco's primary care internal medicine residency. Much of the training was at San Francisco General Hospital, an academic safety-net hospital that attracted Adams as the Bay Area equivalent of Denver Health. The residency embraced evidence-based medicine, a rationalized approach to medical decision-making where a physician employs statistical measures to select her diagnostic and treatment approaches. Most internal medicine residencies embrace evidence-based medicine, but Adams's residency extended its evidence-based approach to medical education, thinking systematically about the best way to train residents to care for the underserved, especially people with HIV. The faculty who trained Adams were part of a chastened generation who had witnessed the HIV epidemic rage through their patient's bodies and communities. In response, the faculty taught a rigorous approach to clinical medicine and medical education. Adams says, simply, that it was "everything I was looking for."

. . .

Today's students are looking for something more like Adams's experience than Osler's day-tight compartments. When she recruits students, Adams calls out the differences to them. "I'm looking for students to partner with me. This is a new model. It's still an experiment, and I am looking for students to improve it with me." She tells them that in Osler's clinical year students rotate at multiple hospitals and clinics, each with their own culture and EHR system. Adams asks them to do something else, saying, "Third year should be about learning clinical medicine, not learning a new EHR every month." She wants students to learn one clinical site, one clinical culture, one EHR and, most importantly, to be educated by one group of patients. "You will have a role in the clinical enterprise, have an authentic role in patient encounters. My students talk about how they can advocate for their patients and help with transitions of care. My students visit their patients in their homes. My students go everywhere in the system with our patients, so they learn it better than many of the faculty, who spend most of their time in their own clinical area."

Adams offers professional relationships, following patients, instead of professional roles, following specialties, as a new way to traverse a complex system. Instead of being passed from attending physician to attending physician every week, they will be assigned to a small group of handpicked teachers for a year. With their core supervising physician, they will see patients each week in the physician's clinic. They will know them well enough to earn a patient's shimmy of approval.

. . .

Mallory and Adams review the afternoon schedule and select the next patient for Mallory to see: Edith.

Edith is no grump but rather an agreeable, older Black woman with salt-and-pepper hair that dances off her head in a soft frizz. She wears red glasses but no makeup that might mask the remarkable adornment of her smile. Mallory has never met her before. Edith sets the tone, even though Mallory asks the first question.

"What would you like to talk about today?

Edith knows a rookie. "I have this odor down here that I don't like." Then she laughs as she says, "It can't be sexual. It's been eleven years."

"Okay, we can take a look. What else?"

Edith tugs at her shirt and says, "I have this mole or blemish."

"Okay, we can look at that. Anything else?"

"I was taking this Restasis for dry eyes. It had a $540 copay. That is way too much. I need something else."

"I don't know who could afford that. We'll try to find something else. I looked over your records. Have you had your flu vaccine?"

"I got it at Walgreens and brought the paper."

"Perfect. What about your shingles vaccine?"

"I got it here, three years ago."

Mallory nods, mentally assuring herself that she has a working problem list for the day's encounter, and begins working through the list.

"What would you like to start with? The odor?"

"Yes. It started a couple of months ago. I don't have any discharge. I think it's just because I'm old," Edith laughingly reports.

"Just the smell. And no intercourse for 11 years."

"Yes, 11 years, can you believe it?"

Mallory reviews Edith's washing regimen. *Dove soap.* She asks after urinary problems. *None.*

"For many of us, a smell can develop because of a yeast infection or a bacterial overgrowth."

"I try to be my own physician. You know, there's nothing cleaning it out down there anymore. I don't know why it's happening. I feel like a young woman. I act like a young woman. I don't want to be smelling like an old woman."

"And what about the blemish?"

"I'm a seventy-year-old woman. I've got nothing to hide."

Unbidden, Edith stands up, takes off her coat, and pulls her heather-gray sweatshirt three-quarters of the way up to reveal a small dark spot underneath her bra on the side of her breast. Mallory palpates it. Borders regular, color uniform. Edith reports no pain on palpation, and Mallory observes no discharge. Mallory reassures her but promises to let Adams know.

As they continue, Mallory reviews medications, but Edith steers them elsewhere, pulling up her sweatshirt to reveal her paunch. She pats it twice and asks, "How can I reduce this," as it jiggles gently. Mallory fumbles a bit, but then she uses Adams's question for herself. "What is the one thing you would like to change about the way you eat?"

"Sweets. In the building I live, there are gatherings. They serve ice cream. I love ice cream. Then they have bake sales with cupcakes every Wednesday. They have fundraisers for our council. So many sweets. Dinners and potlucks. I'm so social I have to be down there."

"I would love to be there too. Ice cream is the best. Could you try fruit instead of the sweets?"

"I could probably do that. When I stayed away from the socials, I lost fifteen pounds, but I'm so social. I want to attend."

They review Edith's medications together and examine her eyes. Then Mallory asks about socializing.

"What about the men where you live?"

"Those are old men. I want a younger man that can keep up with me. They're more fun."

Mallory blushes and smiles, "I agree." The two then share a laugh while Mallory listens to Edith's heart by snaking the stethoscope down the front of her sweatshirt, and then she asks permission to listen to her lungs.

"You know those old men in the apartment complex, they chase me."

"Well, I wish you luck with that. I will talk with Dr. Adams about this and we'll come back with a plan for today."

Mallory departs and finds Adams. They both suspect bacterial vaginosis. Together, they develop a plan to treat Edith: self-swab, treatment if she has bacterial vaginosis, and return visit. If she is still experiencing symptoms at the next visit, they will perform a full pelvic exam. Mallory describes Edith's skin lesion as a non-concerning small blemish. Adams helps her translate her finding into medical language. The blemish becomes a papule without asymmetry, regular borders, uniform dark-brown color, and diameter less than a centimeter.

They return to the room, and Adams takes the lead.

"How've you been doing?"

Edith smiles. "Nice and sassy."

"They told me."

"They told *on* me. Well, now you know that I'm myself."

"I do. I hear you're worried about your weight, but we checked and it's the same as last time. Mallory says you're going to watch your sweets, which is my weakness too."

"Oh, I will. I was coming in today and my son told me to listen to you. You always do a good job of finding out what's wrong with me. I trust you."

Adams asks to see the blemish. Edith stands, pulls up her sweatshirt, and reveals her right breast. Adams examines the papule. She turns to Mallory and says, "I have a diagnosis. Run your finger on it. Does it feel kind of sandpapery?" Mallory rubs her fingertips underneath Edith's bra strap.

"Yes."

"Do you have a diagnosis?"

"Seborrheic keratosis."

"Yes! They often form as we age, especially in places where people have friction, like right along the bra line. Edith, you're going to be okay. There's nothing to do about these."

Edith interrupts the doctor talk with her own interpretation. "There are so many things which happen as you age. I guess this is just one of them."

They continue, but Edith has the last word, shimmying her hips as she tells Mallory and Adams, "I need someone who can keep up with me. Now that I've turned seventy, I want to make changes. I want to live my life."

This is the chance Adams is offering: learn from two textbooks, over time, so that you can earn shimmies. Adams is betting that the LIC—with its small cohort of learners, its sustained engagement with a small number of faculty, and its continuity with patients—is a structure to change medicine. In the nineteenth century, medical students were apprentices. In the twentieth century, the work of physicians like Osler inspired reformers like Flexner, and the resulting training model turned medical students into professionals. Osler and Flexner spoke to their moment, a time when what physicians needed were advances in the basic sciences. We still ask today's med students to follow them into the day-tight compartments from a century ago, even as everything else about medical practice has changed. In the twenty-first century, Adams wants students like Mallory to move at just the right speed to become companions.

Chapter 10

COFFEE SHOP REVOLUTION

JUST A FEW MONTHS into the year, Maggie Kriz is already changing course. "I think I had this idea of who I was and which path I wanted my career to take. Spending time with people has made me realize that other things are more important to me than I necessarily thought." She finds that knowing someone medically is funny because it gets to the core of a person like an intense relationship, but you ask different questions and keep different boundaries. Maggie thinks about those limits when she remembers Kenny, the traveler who became a double amputee while she followed him through his time in the hospital. Maggie stayed to journey with more patients. Kenny left the hospital for home.

"I'm just wondering is it appropriate to call the phone number that he left, obviously, with a blocked number, just to check to see if he made it. I don't know. What boundaries do I draw? Obviously, I would never friend him on Facebook or give him my actual number or my email or anything like that, but I'm curious to know how he's doing and if he's okay. I don't know."

Maggie met Kenny as a student, sharing an intense encounter that altered both of their lives, and it left her wondering if and how she can know him further. She wants to know how he is, how his story ends, but

without sharing her number. Medical knowing is as emotionally intense as a close friendship and as physically intimate as a romance, but
limited by the patient-physician relationship. Maggie finds that while
you can always check in with an old friend, medical stories end when
patient and physician part. As a student still becoming a doctor, medical stories leave Maggie with feelings that blur boundaries. Instead
of acting on those feelings, Maggie works those feelings out in the
classroom.

Next to the LIC classroom, Kristina Oatis keeps an office.
Mounted on the far wall are her many awards for training medical students like Maggie. She is here for those students, but what she keeps
close to her desk is a snapshot of six women at a New Kids on the Block
(NKOTB) concert dressed, like their heroes, in identical outfits. Her
friends call her Kris, and all six of them are wearing tank tops proudly
proclaiming their wearers Blockheads 4 Life. Oatis loves the coordinated costumes, the synchronized steps, and the way Danny, Don-
nie, Joey, Jonathan, and Jordan work together. Oatis spends many
vacations attending NKOTB shows with friends she met on the boy
band circuit. She is here for these women too. Oatis likes teamwork in
motion and has been teaching teamwork as the LIC coordinator since
the program's inception.

When Dr. Adams was dreaming up the LIC, Oatis was working at
the University of Colorado School of Medicine as the student coordinator for the internal medicine clerkship. In the traditional clinical year,
internal medicine typically takes up a full three months. Since Osler,
this has been the cornerstone of the clinical year, but Oatis wonders if it
was crumbling. She felt that students were cycling through too quickly.
"There's no continuity with people. It's these very brief episodes with
them, and I just never felt fulfilled with that." Looking for a better way
to train med students, she was excited when the med school flew in
Dr. David Hirsh for a talk. Oatis listened as Hirsh spoke about the LIC

at Cambridge Health Alliance, a safety-net system affiliated with Harvard Medical School. Oatis says, "It was like lights and bells and whistles and everything went off." Oatis recognized the problems that Hirsh named—disconnection, discouragement, disengagement—in her internal medicine clerkship students, and she thought that his solution was a better way.

When Adams called afterward and asked if Oatis would train the coordinator for a local version of Hirsh's program, Oatis turned the tables. She asked to be hired as the LIC coordinator.

They have been teammates ever since, equally enthusiastic about the work. Oatis loves the LIC. She loves Dr. Adams, but she never calls her that. It is Kris and Jen, Jen and Kris. A duo rather than a full band. They rely on each other even more and share the same affections, including Denver Health.

"I have been a patient at some of the best-known, world-class facilities, where the buildings were all new and the furniture was all new and fancy. And I've been to places where it's not that way. At the end of the day, I don't care if the couch I'm sitting on is brand new, but if the person that's providing me care is dedicated to being there and providing me the best health care possible no matter what my situation is, that is way more important to me."

Oatis and Adams share what NKOTB called a righteous mission. They share not only joy but also anger, especially when someone speaks unfavorably about Denver Health or its patients. Oatis explains, her voice rising, "Somebody who's working with students and says derogatory things about the patient population . . . [or] people here that are going against the mission and everything we stand for, angers Jen to no end."

Oatis's voice rises as she concludes, "There are other places that say obviously their mission is research, education, and health care, but I've never felt it more than I have here."

Oatis makes sure the LIC students feel her care as well. She occupies only a corner of the office, populating the rest of her office with workstations, coffeepots, and chairs—all for the students. It's rare to find Oatis alone in her office. She is usually hosting a student like Maggie who claims to need help with a clinical schedule, or parking, or exams but is waiting for a chance to talk through the feelings of missing a patient like Kenny. Oatis's warm concern makes the space, an awkward L-shaped room, feel like a home.

Oatis makes her own home a few miles from the hospital, with her husband and their dog. She has no kids of her own, so the students play the part, texting her their problems on days and nights, weekdays and weekends. No matter the time, when a student texts, Oatis responds quickly. Each response builds the relationship, and the relationships feel too important to allow her to draw boundaries between work and life. "I get so excited to hear about what they did in their day and what cool LIC things that they got to do today, like planning their next month, and seeing them grow."

In another life, Oatis would see them grow as a colleague. She sometimes imagines being an internist herself, but she dislikes blood and student loans. She feels like she gets the best parts of being a physician, the problem-solving and the relationships. "I tell people, 'I've landed where I'm supposed to.'"

The students come, spend a year haunting her office and texts, and then join the alumni pictures on the classroom's grandmother wall, not far from the needlepoint. The daily relationship that endures is between Kris and Jen, which Oatis credits as resulting from the fact that "we're both doing our jobs because we really want to do our jobs."

Kris and Jen work together, like NKOTB, step by step, planning the students' movements. Kris reads the evaluations of each student experience and alters the students' schedules, dropping teaching physicians who fail to teach and moving lectures to better prepare students for exams. The students, Kris says, trust "that we're really looking out for their future and the best career training possible for them." Step by step, they need each other. They have so much to do for these students, and for the future of medicine.

. . .

Like so many world-altering schemes, the LIC began on a coffee shop napkin. Dr. David Hirsh remembers the powerful paper rectangle he shared with Dr. Barbara Ogur. "We sat in the coffee shop, and we were starting to have this conversation where we were saying we love being doctors. It's such a great thing to be a doctor. It's so meaningful. We were just feeling lucky. And then of course it went on to, 'We love being teachers. We really enjoy our students so much. We feel so lucky.' And then we turned a little pensive, wondering, 'Why don't our students love their clinical year of med school as much as we love being doctors?' We were thinking about all of these students we had known in the pre-clerkship years who were full of gusto, and full of energy, and so idealistic. And then we would meet them sometimes after their core clinical year and they had more fatigue or dismay."

They were watching their students become discouraged and disengaged as they followed Harvard faculty through clerkships in internal medicine, pediatrics, obstetrics, psychiatry, and surgery. As the clinical year went on, the students calloused up, reading less and caring less.

"We didn't want to simply accept that, well, they got older and they saw hard things. Or they are tired. We were wondering why they didn't have that full-hearted, full-throated, intellectual, but also soulful, interest in their patients in the way that we hoped."

Hirsh and Ogur had once followed Flexner's curriculum and Osler's counsel. The journey had built them up. Hirsh became a family practitioner; Ogur, an internist. Both found purposeful work in their ability to form working relationships with patients, to know and be known, in sickness and health. They encouraged students down the same educational path, only to become discouraged when their students felt diminished by the journey. Students found medical training extensive, as subspecialty fellowships can extend a physician's medical training well past a decade, and expensive, with many graduating with half a million dollars in educational debt. Students were so overwhelmed by the many technical elements of the textbook of the body— the sixty-five hundred medical devices a physician could install, the twenty thousand approved medications they could prescribe, the sixty-eight thousand billing codes a physician could use—that they settled for learning instead of forming meaningful relationships with patients [38]. On the napkin, Hirsh and Ogur sketched out a different path for their students.

"We came upon the idea that we had meaningful relationships with our patients and we had meaningful roles with our patients. Our patients seemed to be counting on us. And if we didn't know something, we had to go read about it, or study it, or figure it out for them, or find the resource. So, what we were thinking is, 'Our students deserve to have that level of uplift, even as they are learning. We have this intellectual curiosity, or wonder, that can play out when we see our patients. We can act upon our wonder, and our wonder is derived from the duty and commitment driving our learning."

They recognized that it is a great small grace to live a life in which you are the one who is kind. They sought a way for their students to experience small graces, to form relationships with both patients and colleagues. "We would miss our patients if they were to move. And if we were even having a chance to be kind towards our patients, being kind felt happy-making."

On the napkin, they worked out a plan to transform medical education through continuity: medical students would follow patients over their clinical year, accompanying them in operating rooms, clinics, and emergency departments, regardless of specialty. To restore the mean-ingful experiences Hirsh and Ogur were after, they wanted students to try on many different roles.

In any teaching hospital, you can chart three simple roles: student, patient, and teacher. But within those categories, many potential sub-roles are played. Spend time with a stack of thesauruses—some find it telling that Peter Mark Roget began his famous one while training young physicians as a faculty surgeon—and you can imagine different roles for students, just like Hirsh and Ogur did [39].

Roles for students: Abecedarian. Amateur. Apprentice. Bonesetter. Cadet. Catechumen. Collaborator. Colt. Convert. Disciple. Docent. Fledgling. Greenhorn. Gremlin. Neophyte. Novice. Protégé. Pupil. Re-cruit. Registrant. Rookie. Servant. Tyro.

Roles for patients: Chump. Client. Consumer. Consumptive. Con-valescent. Customer. Dependent. Incurable. Neighbor. Patron. Shop-per. Shut-In. Sufferer. Textbook. Walk-In. Ward.

Roles for teachers: Coach. Evaluator. Faculty. Gradgrind. Lecturer. Master. Mentor. Overseer. Pedant. Preceptor. Scholar. Supervisor.

So many roles to pick from, each emphasizing different aspects of learning, receiving care, and instructing. The role you pick shapes how students like Maggie can meet patients like Kenny while being taught by physicians like Adams.

That day in the coffee shop, Hirsh and Ogur decided that stu-dents, patients, and teachers needed a structure for medical knowing. After exploring all the learning and caregiving roles, they decided that students should be companions. Not just people who watched the ill, but people who participated in their care, even their lives. It was, after all, a common thread: students, patients, and teachers could all accompany each other as they cared for others.

Hirsh recalls, "I mean, we call them 'teachers,' or 'preceptors,' but we faculty don't always have preceptors watching us or grading us. We have colleagues whom we feel close to and are excited to be with. So why couldn't students have their preceptor, or their overseer, or their guide, or their coach, or role model be someone they were excited to go see?

"The whole notion was to reconstitute relationships and to have meaningful roles. Meaningful roles vis-à-vis the teacher. Meaningful roles vis-à-vis most importantly the patient. And what would the educational structure be like to do that? Our first thought was we should redesign the internal medicine clerkship to be longitudinal and do a pilot of that.

"And then our next thought was, 'Maybe we should redesign the entire year.' Because we were thinking about things like, 'Can you imagine if you could see patients in surgery before you knew if they needed a surgery? And then you could see them in the surgery. And then you could see them after the surgery. And then you could see them in some other venue, when it wasn't surgical at all.'

"Because after somebody has their gallbladder taken out, they are still a person who might need health care in other ways or who has mental health needs not as a consequence of the surgery. Why couldn't you see them for mental health needs too? Why couldn't you learn longitudinally across the venues, across the disciplines, and try to reconstitute holistic understandings of people? Or watching a child develop over one year, or being there for someone's entire pregnancy and then delivering them, and then taking care of the child, and then seeing them again as a now non-pregnant adult needing health care?

"So those things led us to a structure that would have the chance to have relationships changed and roles changed. Meaningful roles. Duty and commitment would drive the learning. And they would be close to their patients and to their teachers."

. . .

Maggie was making her way down the coffee shop path charted by Hirsh and Ogur.

"I'm one of those people who just feels all the feels. I've talked to Mackenzie and there are some things that I feel have really affected me in really strong ways and other things that I thought would affect me in really strong ways did not. I'm still getting used to it. It seems like there's like no clear pattern. When I'm going to cry and when I'm not going to cry and when I'm going to be fine. I really like to talk about things and oftentimes will discuss my feelings about what I've seen, without going into too much detail, with my friends and family. But in a lot of ways, I don't tell them a lot of stuff because I think 'I'm the one who signed up for this and I don't really want to put this on you.'"

When she does confide in them, Maggie finds it hard to explain to her friends and family what is happening. She can tell stories, but only without identifying details, so the stories are difficult to understand. Details are what make stories real. Medical details are both private and technical, making them doubly difficult for someone outside medicine to fully understand. Sometimes you settle for an impression instead of a story.

"I do tell occasional stories, you know, when something really exciting has happened and they're just always, 'You have the craziest job in the world.' And I say, 'Yeah. I do. It's insane.' Really amazing."

Maggie, like her classmates, is still figuring out her relationship to the people she meets as patients and how to tell her friends and family about her work. Sometimes it leaves her feeling lonely, sometimes joyful, sometimes sad—all the feels you get from drawing close to the ill.

. . .

To account for that closeness, those relationships students have with their patients and their teachers, Hirsh likes to cite another Progressive Era reformer, John Dewey, as an inspiration for the LIC. In *Education and Experience*, Dewey wrote, "The two principles of continuity and interaction are not separate from each other. They intercept and unite. They are, so to speak, the longitudinal and lateral aspects of experience.

Different situations succeed one another. But because of the principle of continuity something is carried over the earlier to the later ones" [40, p. 44].

So when Hirsh and Ogur finally announced the LIC to the medical world, they did so in a paper entitled "'Continuity' as an Organizing Principle for Clinical Education Reform." In medical journalese, they were signaling that their idea was not just another curriculum but a true reform, a way to make companions out of the students, patients, and teachers moving together through the strange worlds of medicine. With Dewey, they believed that education should be active and relational.

It had only taken them four years to advance from a coffee shop napkin to announcing a call for reform from the pages of the *New England Journal of Medicine*. They wrote, "Continuity of care provides students with relevant, extended, and serial contact with patients, physician preceptors, and other health care professionals. The goals of students and patients are aligned, and students become natural advocates for their patients' interests and needs" [41, p. 864]. If a student were to have continuity of care, continuity of curriculum, and continuity of supervision, they could experience a continuity of idealism. Those were the steps to becoming companions.

Hirsh and Ogur wanted to help all the people—patient, student, teacher—involved in clinical encounters. They worked at Cambridge Health Alliance, a safety-net system affiliated with the ivoriest of ivory towers, Harvard Medical School. Even there, they found that the pace of today's medicine was too fast to teach, and most of the faculty were tasked with producing clinical outcomes instead of getting to know their students and patients.

So Hirsh and Ogur recruited faculty and randomized eight Harvard medical students to help them develop a new dance. The steps went like this: every week, each student spent a half day in their supervising physicians' clinics. In these clinics, the faculty and students selected patients together. They sought patients with the major diseases and presentations every future doctor should know. Then the students followed their patients through the system. They received electronic alerts when one of their patients was hospitalized.

At 7:00 a.m., a student rounded on her hospitalized patients, visiting each patient to assess their medical progress as part of a teaching team of resident and attending physicians. By 9:00 a.m., a student joined her supervising physician in clinic. In the afternoons, if not in clinic, she read or attended case-based tutorials, learning with her fellow LIC students, or checked up on patients by phone. By 5:00 p.m., a student rounded again on any of her patients who were hospitalized.

Some weeks, a student immersed herself in surgery, but even then, she kept up her relationship with her core teacher, her core patients, and her classmates. Hirsh and Ogur surveyed and assessed the students and faculty; they found the experience to be more hectic but more humanizing than the traditional clinical year. Students accompanied patients through an entire course of illness, from initial concern in a clinic, to evaluation in an emergency department, to hospitalization on the wards, to discharge home. On these journeys, Hirsh and Ogur regained their hope for medical education, writing that these longitudinal students may "become agents of change for a return to a more effective, humanistic, and fulfilling practice of medicine" [42, p. 403].

Only six years post-napkin, Hirsh and Ogur and their colleagues began publishing the LIC's benefits. LIC students were more patient centered, more likely to enter primary care, more likely to report mentoring relationships, and more likely to encounter the everyday health conditions prevalent in a community instead of the rare cases found in hospital clerkships at quaternary care medical centers [43].

When they published outcome data, they reported that LIC students were, with the help of someone like Oatis keeping them in step, seeing patients before, during, and after an episode of acute illness and were almost twice as likely to form meaningful relationships with patients. A dean at the medical school expressed surprise at how much better Hirsh and Ogur found their program to be, so Hirsh titled their next paper "Better Learning, Better Doctors, Better Delivery System." They reported that LIC students received more feedback and better mentoring from faculty [44]. Better meant betterment, Hirsh was saying to the dean. He kept on, finding that the LIC improves student communication skills, increases clinical reasoning, helps students become patient centered and community minded, and results in better student satisfaction than traditional clerkships, all while achieving at least equivalent examination scores [45]. And the effect endured. When they surveyed LIC alumni four to six years after graduation, the LIC students were more likely to be self-reflective, to involve patients in decision-making, to relate to people across their life span, to understand how their social context affected their health, and to be their patients' advocates. A single year in the LIC kept physicians engaged with their patients for years afterward [46].

Buoyed by their results, Hirsh and Ogur shared them with colleagues around the world. They found evidence that educators had trialed continuity before—Case Western had piloted longitudinal care that bridged obstetrics and pediatrics, and the rural track of a Minnesota medical school began longitudinal training all the way back in 1971—and the idea had spread, but only to a handful of rural schools. Rural communities embraced the LIC both because they lacked the strata of researchers and subspecialists who populate an academic medical center and because training medical students in rural communities increased the odds that they would practice in rural communities [47].

Just like the world conquerors in NKTOB, Hirsh and Ogur had ambitions beyond niche status. For better or worse, ideas spread faster from Harvard than from Minnesota. They knew that while Flexner had advanced Osler's curriculum without any hard evidence that it produced better doctors, it had become accepted wisdom. In the century since, there had been cycle after cycle of curriculum reform [48, 49, 50, 51], but most resulted in variations on Osler's curriculum. It all amounted to what, in 1989, the medical sociologist S. W. Bloom called "reform without change," because the changes never challenged what he called "the way the complex modern corporate bureaucracy is experienced by new doctors" and how it resists "community-oriented problem-based learning" [52, p. 238]. Curriculum innovations never changed the existential core of the Oslerian curriculum, which tied medical training and practice to research-based universities and the meritocrats who populated them, because they never really changed the culture of medicine. And even though all these variations to the customary clinical year lacked evidence, just like the original Oslerian model, medical school deans were accustomed to the typical training model. The typical version resembled their own training and supported the existing medical hierarchy, so the deans raised skeptical queries whenever a true reform was discussed, even when evidence showed the benefits of problem-based and collaborative learning models [13]. To win over skeptics, Hirsh and Ogur set out to assess the LIC, eventually publishing so widely that the LIC has become the most evidence based of all medical curricula. Hirsh and Ogur spread the word in journals and at conferences. They found believers. Some medical schools—like University of California, San Francisco, where Adams completed residency—added LIC tracks. Now, medical students in Australia, Canada, Ireland, New Zealand, Norway, Singapore, South Africa, and the United Kingdom are being educated in LICs [53], and the number of LICs is growing [54].

Hirsh and Ogur have company, so they and their colleagues study variations of the model from around the world. LICs can be either a track within the curriculum or the curriculum itself. LICs can last two years instead of one [55]. LICs can work in rural or urban settings. LICs can work in both community health settings and tertiary academic medical centers [56, 57].

There are so many variations that Hirsh and his colleagues developed a typology. There are rural LICs, where primary care physicians were more prevalent, and urban LICs, where subspecialists play a larger role in the training. There are amalgamations with traditional clerkships, in which students spent less than half of their clinical year in an LIC. There are blended programs, in which students spend a portion of their clinical year in an LIC. And there are comprehensive programs, in which a student's entire clinical year is a longitudinal, integrated experience [58].

The idea changes at each site, such as the adaptation designed by local duo Kris and Jen, but Hirsh and Ogur observe that three core principles endure through every adaptation: students need a meaningful role in continually caring for a group of patients, a continuous learning relationship with teachers, and sufficient experiences in multiple disciplines to meet the core clinical competencies [59]. Providing these essentials can make for better doctors and more socially accountable medical schools [60]. As LIC students participate in the comprehensive care of patients over time, through continuous relationships with preceptors and the community, Hirsh declares, medical education can once again be a social good. The LIC is a way to train physicians who have Ogur's joy for medicine and are connected to their patients, their peers, their preceptors, and the public.

Hirsh and Ogur sometimes argue that the LIC is also a return to what Flexner sought in the first place. They like to quote from the *Flexner Report* itself: "To sample a school on its clinical side, one makes in the first place straight for its medical clinic, seeking to learn the number of patients available for teaching, the variety of conditions that they illustrate, and the hospital regulations in so far, at least, as they determine (1) continuity of service on the part of the teachers of medicine, (2) the closeness that the student may follow the individual patients . . ." [44, p. 649]. Hirsh and Ogur want to restore the continuity of service and the closeness of students to individual patients for a different health care structure.

When Hirsh tells medical educators about the LIC, quoting Flexner is reassuring. It also elides the differences between the Flexnerian and LIC models. The final item on Flexner's list of what medical training needed was "(3) the access of the student to the clinical laboratory" [14, p. 94]. When Flexner wrote of continuity, he often meant a continuity between medical training and scientific inquiry, but the LIC does not require a laboratory to drive scientific discovery. The LIC requires human connections to drive humane inquiry. That very much includes science, but Hirsh and Ogur value curiosity and connection in all its forms over any particular learning activity. "It's a way of animating the human heart," Hirsh says, "to drive curiosity."

To incite that curiosity in service of others, Hirsh likes to use an old-fashioned bit of poetry, Tennyson's "Ulysses." When he visits med schools to spread the word about the LIC, he usually recites the last stanza, where Tennyson assures his friends that it is "not too late to seek a newer world," and concludes that, like the poet's protagonist, they must set out "to strive, to seek, to find, and not to yield" [61, p. 71].

As it happens, Dewey quoted the same poem in *Experience and Education*, but Dewey preferred an earlier stanza: "all experience is an arch wherethro' / Gleams that untravell'd world whose margin fades / Forever and forever when I move." Experience is like an arch that, after passing through it, changes how you are in the world.

Today's medical educators know that it matters with whom you pass through the arch. Oatis sometimes wonders if boy-band-level discipline, not Tennyson or Dewey, is what we need today. Boy bands have stable teams that train together for years before they hang tough together in a performative environment. Boy bands have managers and techs to make sure they hit every mark on their state-of-the-art stage. They have a Svengali manager and corporate sponsorship.

Kris and Jen have no Svengali or sponsor. They partner with a leading medical school, but they work at a perpetually underfunded safety-net hospital that is forever passing the proverbial hat to raise funds. They don't have a fancy stage, but salvaged furniture from the past century. It's more like busking. They don't have a crew; they have each other.

Step by step / Don't you know I need you.

They also have the LIC students, whom Kris and Jen are turning into a team. The students are the true new kids, but together they are becoming physicians and then, Kris and Jen hope, teachers themselves. They need to follow the steps on the coffeehouse napkin, wherever they lead.

. . .

Maggie was making her way down the path charted by Hirsh and Ogur. She had felt that closeness with patients like Kenny. Every time she thinks of him, she tears up. "There's this guy who's literally the same age as me who had a similar life and just through a series of unfortunate events . . ." She trails off into tears, but then continues, "I miss him. He's still homeless. Even though I've never experienced homelessness, I worked 40 hours a week, I worked overnights with people experiencing homelessness or three overnights a week in [the shelters]." Maggie pauses, remembering Kenny and the people experiencing homelessness that she has known. "I've seen how hard that life is. Not only is he homeless and an IV drug user, but he has no legs." Maggie continues to reminisce about Kenny. "He was a musician and had another tattoo with some lyrics from a song that he wrote. And I asked, 'Do you play guitar anymore?' He showed me his hand, which I hadn't noticed before, but it was permanently stuck." Looking closely, Maggie saw that Kenny's fingers, harmed by infections and injections, could no longer move well enough to play guitar, but he could offer his hand for her examination and care. Maggie could take Kenny's hand in her own and then remember that feeling, step by step, as she became a doctor.

Chapter 11

DOWNWARD ARROW

*A*S MACKENZIE GARCIA FOLLOWED HER PATIENTS, she felt herself going down dangerous paths. It started early, on her first twenty-four-hour trauma surgery shift. An MVC—motor vehicle crash—presented to the trauma bay. She was one of two students on trauma, but there was room for only one of them at the operating table. The other med student scrubbed in; Mackenzie watched for hours as the surgeons reassembled jigsawed bodies.

"I had a very strong emotional reaction to it. I don't know why I didn't anticipate that. I have a therapist. I talked about anticipating other things, but for some reason I hadn't particularly anticipated what I would encounter on trauma surgery. I had two cousins die when I was ten and then eleven. One died in a car crash, and then one was shot in the head. So, I don't know why in my mind I didn't think, 'Oh, getting shot and car crashes are the most common trauma surgery things.'"

After the case, after the surgical day turned into a surgical night and another surgical day, Mackenzie left the hospital only to attend the funeral of a friend who had lost his own battle with cancer. It was the kind of day where all you see is loss and all you feel is down.

. . .

In therapy, a therapist can teach you how to control a downward descent. The therapist can teach you why some experiences take you down and where those experiences lead you. The therapist shows you that those experiences lead to what you deeply believe. To get you there, the therapist can employ the downward arrow technique. You tell the therapist an automatic thought. *I should have anticipated that I would see car crashes and gunshot wounds on trauma surgery.* The therapist asks you how the automatic thought felt and what it would mean if this thought were true. *Why should you have anticipated someone else's work?* Each time you answer. *I should have known better.* The therapist digs down, layer after layer, until you disclose a belief about who you are. *I fail those who die on my watch.*

The downward arrow travels to the beliefs holding you captive [62].

. . .

Just a few days before, Mackenzie had felt good, even energized. She was on the internal medicine wards, and it felt like her team. She liked the work of untangling a patients' acute problems from chronic ailments. She liked the organizing of illness into detailed, hierarchical problem lists and then addressing each numbered problem daily. She liked the detective work, which felt like learning "what happened in a person's life to get them to this point and what will happen to them in the future." After her brief rotation, she wanted to follow the patients longer, to untangle their problems down to the systemic level. Internal medicine felt like it could be the specialty for her.

Surgery felt different. She began her four-week surgery immersion with a cold that felt like a physical manifestation of her cooling expectations for the specialty. The patients were the same, but the team engaged them differently. Surgeons harmed to heal. They knew most of their patients for a short time. Their time together was intensely intimate, at least physically. And the actions they undertook would be criminal outside of the operating room, cutting open the body and removing or altering its insides. Mackenzie often found herself asking different questions than the surgeons. If she identified wheezing on a pulmonary examination and asked, "Shouldn't we do something about that?" she would hear, "That's not something we do something about." The surgeons focused on the acute somethings: the car crashes and cancers.

Mackenzie always felt out of phase on surgery. On her first day, she ran to catch up with surgeons as they went into the OR. It was a six-hour case, and she couldn't leave to eat or use the bathroom. "I got light-headed, and the scrub tech had to tape my glasses onto my hat because they kept falling down because I didn't have my Croakies thing. It was sort of a mess."

The attending surgeon on the case was Dr. Kshama Jaiswal, the breast surgeon with the queen-size coffee mug. The case was a double mastectomy for a woman in her seventies, a meticulous operation in which Jaiswal had to account for dozens of blood vessels. Jaiswal proceeded at a gradual pace, using a Bovie knife, an electric knife that uses high-frequency oscillations to cut cancers or coagulate capillaries.

Mackenzie thinks that the light-headedness was probably due in part to the Bovie. "There's a lot of Bovie in mastectomies, burning the tissue, and so it is very smelly in a way that I had not anticipated—the burning smell of flesh."

Jaiswal saw Mackenzie looking woozy and motioned to the circulating nurse, who brought her a stool. She scrubbed out, drank some water, and then returned. This time, a nurse taped the bridge of Mackenzie's eyeglasses to her forehead and covered it all with a scrub cap before sending her back to the operating theater.

Mackenzie came back prepared for the smell and the impersonal nature of surgery. The blue sheet was draped around the patient so that only the anesthesiologist could see her face, and with another sheet draped around her legs and abdomen, only the chest was exposed. It was a controlled context—she never met the patient outside the operating room—and Mackenzie steadied herself by thinking, "This is helping this person, it's not hurting them."

For her next few days on surgery, Mackenzie focused simply on not accidentally hurting anyone. She found that she could begin "trying to understand what's going on, trying to see the anatomy when I'm able to, trying to follow the surgical decision-making that's going on."

. . .

A couple of months before Mackenzie's first day on surgery, Dr. Adams concluded orientation by warning the students of the three Ds to which they could succumb: *depression, divorce,* and *drink.* All three were more likely for physicians than the average person with their educational level. All three needed to be resisted daily through habits that helped a doctor survive. Adams ended orientation with a warning: "You need to start developing these lifelong skills as third years, because it doesn't get easier. Fourth year has its challenges. Residency is hard. Being an attending is hard."

Privately, Adams admitted that it sometimes seemed too hard. She felt like every female physician she knew was taking an antidepressant. She recalled residents who left training programs because of the stress. She remembered students who missed clinical days, only to be discovered in their closed garage, running their car engine, and wondering how much exhaust it would take to end their own life. Thinking of these students, residents, and faculty, Adams cried and asked, "What's wrong with this profession? What does it mean to recruit students into this when it causes them so much pain?" The questions kept her up at night. She feared the day when one of her students, who had learned exactly how much exhaust will suffocate, how many pills to swallow, which vessel to slice, would use their textbook-of-the-body knowledge to fatally exit the field. She could not believe that medical training and practice had to be this way.

Even worse, Adams knew that medicine is the only advanced degree that increases a person's chance of dying by suicide. For most people, the more education you get, the lower the chances you will die by suicide; medicine is the exception. While most suicides are associated with an interpersonal crisis, the approximately three hundred physician suicides every year in the United States are more often associated with a work crisis. Physicians identify so deeply with their work that when they experience a work crisis, it can cost them their lives [63, 64].

There is, tragically, another way in which medicine is exceptional. Generally, men die by suicide at a higher rate than women, primarily because men select lethal means for an attempt. And yet female physicians are more likely than male physicians to die by suicide, even when controlling for the specialty they select [65]. Medical training changes your odds. Adams believes that the LIC is part of the solution but worries that it is not enough.

Publicly, she tells the students about healing circles run by an emergency medicine physician, about a morning meditation training program run by a trauma surgeon, about a student mental health day planned for each fall. She hands out an article that argues that the real treatment for physician burnout is collective action [66]. The idea resonates with Adams. Organizing seems, to her, like the next step beyond antidepressants and therapy and resiliency, toward an enduring solution to burnout, a problem facing physicians around the world. She wants to change the confining structures, the day-tight compartments, of a physician's life. She does not want any of her students or residents or faculty to be stuck inside their garage, plotting suicide. It is one of her great fears, to lose a trainee or a colleague.

Some resident physicians believe that the solution is joining a formal union. Fifteen percent of the nation's resident physicians already belong to a union, far more than the percentage of practicing physicians, and the number is growing. They hope unionization will renew the profession. A union can negotiate stipends, secure additional benefits, and change clinical schedules for resident physicians. A union cannot address academic issues or alter accreditation standards or compel hospitals to care for the uninsured and the undocumented.

So Adams has not joined a union. She is, like most physicians, a pragmatic problem solver. She is building an educational structure that enables students to flourish, providing relationships to sustain them and support when they feel run down. She informs students of the mental health clinic the medical school organizes. The clinic provides meds—those ubiquitous antidepressants—and therapy for the discouraged and the depressed because the school knows that the work can take you down dangerous paths.

. . .

Caroline Elton, a British vocational psychologist, spent two decades listening to hundreds of medical students and physicians. Elton learned that while medical practice had been transformed—life-prolonging treatments, time-consuming EHRs, ever-increasing operational pressures, inflation-exceeding educational debt—medical training still followed the path drawn up by Osler and prescribed by Flexner, sending students like Mackenzie through research universities and teaching hospitals.

There was one change, however: today's trainees are increasingly isolated. During Adams's training, trainees worked long hours, but they worked them together. Even on nights, teams at academic medical centers often included medical students, interns, residents, and fellows. The day team was sleeping, the visitors had returned home, but the hospital was awake and being run by teams of young people figuring out how to care for the ill together. The introduction of duty hour regulations limited the length and number of overnight shifts without changing the need for someone to work overnight. A generation later, residents now often work nights alone, caring for more patients who are sicker and receiving more complicated treatments, to perform more complex work in more concentrated periods of time. Residents used to follow a patient during the day, when the whole team could see the patient together, and then extend the care into the night. Now they typically come in just for the nights, taking over the care of patients the day team hands off to them. While it means less time in the hospital for many residents and their medical students, it also makes their time in the hospital more isolating. When a resident or student becomes discouraged or overwhelmed by their clinical work, it often happens when they are alone. When they report it to senior physicians, it is often perceived as a failure of empathy instead of acts of self-defense. Elton believes that doctors-in-training activate those psychological defenses as a kind of empathy. A student's distressing tasks eventually remind her that she herself, or her family or friends, could become just as ill.

Patients, Elton observes, can evoke emotional responses from physicians for many reasons, but the deep, core reason is that patients remind physicians that they and all those they love are mortal, will suffer illness or injury, and, despite all the advances of medicine, will eventually die. Since this will inevitably occur during a physician's training and practice—every physician will eventually experience downward arrows that take them to existential questions—Elton argues that we need to assess and bolster emotional resilience. She favors designing a physician's days and nights so they can face, rather than simply feel, the existential questions they confront [67].

. . .

A student like Mackenzie can experience a range of emotions when confronting existential questions. Psychiatrists have correlated which feels students experience with the specialty they select: surgical trainees tend to report experiencing emotional exhaustion, while nonsurgical trainees tend to report experiencing a diminished sense of personal accomplishment [68]. Surgeons feel tired; other physicians feel ineffective.

Even future psychiatrists activate defense mechanisms, but often by intellectualizing all the different ways to conceptualize down feelings. They think about feeling bad, blue, brokenhearted, crestfallen, dejected, despondent, disconsolate, doleful, down in the mouth, downhearted, downcast, gloomy, glum, hangdog, heartsick, melancholic, miserable, sad, sorrowful, woebegone, and wretched. They learn some of the many words to describe these states and the ways different cultures, inside and outside of medicine, conceptualize distress differently. They know that Americans like to talk about burnout, the exhaustion of a machine's finite energy source [69]. Germans talk of entering *Bewusstseinslage*, a state of consciousness devoid of sensory components. Brits talk of losing the bubble, a submariner's term for cracking up while living a constrained life.

And yet the psychiatric research is less colorful, preferring empathy scales to chart the downward decline. Such studies find that medical students often experience a decline of empathy during their clinical training [70], and that decline affects which specialties they enter. The more their vicarious empathy declines, the less likely they are to become a primary care physician like Adams [71]. And even if they manage to follow Adams's path, primary care physicians burn out sooner than their peers despite fewer years of training.

Mackenzie is determined to stay in the field, so she sees a therapist who helps her limn the limits of a physician's work.

"She helped me think that it's almost selfish to think that you can take everything on and solve everything for everyone. That's assuming I have all the answers and then I decide what is best for that person, as opposed to helping them decide on their own. My role is to be supportive and help them get *there* and help them achieve *that* and try to remove barriers that are beyond their control, as much as I can. Ultimately, I got to that point where I gave myself permission to not be the sole carrier of everyone's problems. That took a while, but since I've given myself that permission, it's been helpful."

. . .

A few days later on the trauma surgery service, Mackenzie is in the surgical ICU, observing again, as a resident teaches how to place a chest tube. *Feel for the intercostal space. Make a 2-3 cm incision transversely over the rib. Apply steady pressure over the chest wall over the rib until you are through the parietal pleura. You will hear a pop. Spread the track with your finger. Sweep the chest wall. Guide the chest wall down the track, over the rib, and into the lung. Advance the tube all the way into the lung. Attach it to the Christmas tree adapter. Sew it in. Some people use U stiches; others, anchor stitches.* Trauma pagers beep her team away from the bedside and to the emergency department's trauma bay. She spends the night in the trauma bay and the OR. It is not as organized or as explained as the resident's lesson, but a constant back-and-forth of scissors on skin, scalpel on muscle, and saw on bone.

For Mackenzie, this was the case that took her to the very heart of it all.

. . .

Back in the classroom, Dr. Adams welcomes an avuncular white-haired physician, the Irish American rheumatologist Dr. Dennis Boyle, to share what he thinks is helpful as the downward arrow takes a physician off her path. He queues up his talk. The first slide reads, "Healing the Healer." Boyle begins by asking everyone in the room to stand up. As he reads off symptoms of burnout, he asks people to sit down if they experience the symptom.

You try to be everything for everybody.

Adams sits down. So do Megan Kalata, Mallory Myers, and Itzam Marin.

At the end of a hard day, you feel you haven't made a difference.

A couple more students sit.

You feel like your work is not recognized.

Maggie Kriz and Sarah Bardwell sit.

You feel so strongly about work that you lack a work-life balance.

The whole room is sitting by this point, but Boyle continues.

You feel you have no control over work.

You work in health care.

Now that the students are personally invested, Boyle begins teaching. Burnout, he says, was first studied in safety-net clinical settings like Denver Health. "Burnout seems to be a part of our work at places like this, to be part of the human condition here." Boyle should know, after practicing at Denver Health for decades and teaching for generations.

He summarizes national data while weaving personal stories into his craic. Most of the data, Boyle tells the students, were created by the work groups of Dr. Tait Shanafelt. Shanafelt found that med school was a distressing time for many students and often eroded their mental and physical health [72]. Shanafelt and his colleagues sent out surveys to broad samples of American medical students; over half of the students who completed the entire survey reported burnout. And the students who reported burnout were more likely to endorse less altruistic ideas and admit that they had engaged in unprofessional behavior [73]. Boyle observes that 10 percent of medical students report suicidal ideation [74], and he summarizes, "We lose the equivalent of two classes of medical students each year to suicide." The students sit in silence for a moment.

Boyle returns to the data, observing that Shanafelt and his colleagues eventually conducted even larger studies of practicing physicians. They found that American physicians were more likely to report symptoms of burnout than other workers, that the rates were growing to over half of all physicians, and that it was most prevalent among frontline physicians, those who worked directly with patients, like emergency and primary care physicians [63, 64].

Boyle pauses before confiding that, a quarter century ago, he taught Shanafelt as a University of Colorado medical student, in a small group setting like today's meeting. His former student had made good. Boyle wonders what these students will eventually add to the practice. To illustrate their journey, he shows a picture of a string of hikers, gradually making their way up Mt. Everest. Boyle asks, "Why is it so hard to climb your own mountain?"

Mackenzie says, "Fear of all the examinations and assessment and failure."

Itzam says, "Uncertainty and not knowing where this leads."

"Debt," says Sarah.

Boyle acknowledges their answers but then confides that med school cost $500 a semester when he was a student. The students groan and laugh darkly at the generational discontinuity.

Maggie sees a continuity and asks if burnout is really a new problem or just a new conversation. Dr. Boyle responds that while the data cannot answer that question, he has seen profound change over his career. Only two-thirds of practicing physicians would become a physician again, and 90 percent of physicians would caution a young person about entering the career. A physician's sense of autonomy and sense of purpose have both gone down.

Mackenzie observes that physicians become discouraged by the time spent documenting in the EHR. On cue, Boyle shows a slide of nuns teaching typing and jokes, "I should have taken Sister Mary Jane's typing course." Itzam volunteers that he did, in fact, learn typing from nuns in Mexico. Boyle nods and then shows a picture of his own medical records from his childhood: thirteen years of treatment, and the resulting documentation filled up a single handwritten page. "It's not so much that today's electronic medical record is the problem, it's the amount of time it takes and that you can document at any time. A good doctor can stay up until midnight documenting." In Boyle's era, the medical record stayed at the hospital with the patient, while today's physicians can access the EHR at great physical distance from the patient, so they can document anytime and anywhere.

The students push back a bit. Maggie, in between the peaceful throws she makes of the knitting needles in her hands, which are turning a ball of pink yarn into a winter hat for her brother, says, "I spend some time in the jails. And all the charts are on paper there. You cannot read anything. You cannot find any information. I think that is worse than the electronic health records."

Boyle acknowledges the trade-offs with a knowing nod, then moves on, teaching the students the serenity prayer and its plea for wisdom to know the difference between what you can and cannot change. He shows them the word *docere*, the Latin root for doctor. Boyle asks, "What does 'doctor' mean?"

Mallory, the student of Lady Philosophy, answers, "Teacher."

"That's right and that's one of the joys of medicine. We love having you in the LIC because we get to teach you. And you'll get to teach others yourself. It's one of the pleasures of this life. The joy of being a doctor is the relationships. It's forming close relationships. Life is a journey. Have fun doing it. Take care of each other while doing it."

Boyle, the Hibernian philosopher physician from another generation, departs.

. . .

Mackenzie reflects on the patient she met in the trauma bay.

"He was hit by a car yesterday. Today, I still don't think they know his name, but he was sort of doing okay in the trauma bay, and then his heart stopped, so they did a thoracotomy."

Thoracotomy is the medical way of saying that the surgeons flayed open his chest after the man's pulses vanished under the surgeon's fingers.

"I was just hanging out in the hallway, and the attending called, 'Get the medical student.' I was running in there and trying to get my gloves on; I didn't know what he was going to have me do."

At the surgeon's invitation, Mackenzie reached into the man's open chest and massaged his stalled heart.

"I touched it. It didn't break, which is sort of obvious when you think about it, but in that moment, I was thinking, 'I'm going to mess something up.'"

But her second thought affirmed why she was drawn to medicine in the first place: "It was very cool. Emotionally intense, but mainly really cool. The first time I saw a cadaver, I cried because I thought it was super-awesome and just . . . beautiful, you know?"

So, as she massaged the heart she felt both a twinge of fear—"Oh my God, why are you having me do this in the middle of this trauma? I should probably be out of the way"—and a sense of profundity.

Mackenzie held a heart in her hands, then she gave it back to the resident as the team moved the man from the emergency department to the operating room. For the next two and a half hours they worked on him, diligently searching for the sheared vessels of the injured stranger.

"The whole time they were like, 'We're not sure he's going to make it.'" Though the situation was dire, it was controlled. The surgeons had put a clamp on the aorta, staunching the bleeding. "Since there wasn't active bleeding, it was a little bit calmer, and they were like, 'Okay, we're going to try pressors, we're going to try something else.'" The surgeons tried everything and invited Mackenzie to try with them.

"They actually had me inject epinephrine into the heart, which I did not know was a real thing. I thought that was just a *Pulp Fiction* thing."

"The heart's beating, so it's sort of hard to aim exactly, but you don't have to aim as precisely as you would other things, because it's a big space. And then you pull back to make sure you have blood, to make sure you're in there, and then just inject it."

While Mackenzie worked the heart, others attended to the rest of the body.

"The ortho team opened the pelvis and packed the pelvis. Then they did a chest tube. Then they wanted to make sure there wasn't bleeding from somewhere that they didn't see on the ultrasound, so they did a laparotomy. So, pretty much everything."

Mackenzie admired their everything, their hours of coordinated work wielding brave utensils with skill and fortitude. She was awed by injecting epinephrine directly into the left ventricle, using her hands to inject into what they had previously massaged. And yet, in the usual story of man versus car, the car won again.

"There wasn't anything they could really fix. They kept opening things, but there wasn't that much that they could do, in the end."

The next day's newspaper ran a few inches reporting a traffic fatality overnight. They did not report the dead man's name. Mackenzie did not know it either. What she knew was what his heart felt like when she massaged it, when she injected epinephrine into it, and when it stopped beating. Medical training is often like that, the very feel of death, with a dying person you barely know. Feeling without knowledge, a life turning into a death. Death is the unnamed fourth D lurking behind the three Ds Adams had named, the final material reality behind depression, divorce, and drink.

Mackenzie likes the complicated problems of material realities. She is half-considering psychiatry, but it does not seem material enough to her. She feels drawn to the ways medical problems are often social problems. She thinks often about the social determinants of health—the ways class, race, gender, religion, and other factors determine health outcomes, and the ways homelessness, food insecurity, poverty, racism, misogyny, and xenophobia sicken people. She admires surgery but will decide against it, because the work is indirectly about social determinants.

"In the OR itself, although social determinants might be relevant in the grand scheme of things, the most important thing is what you're doing in that moment." Only if the patient makes it through that moment could the doctor address the other things, which is partially why Mackenzie didn't feel like she fit in with the OR, even as she admired surgeons like Jaiswal and the way they approached patients. Mackenzie knew that the surgeons maintained a certain clinical distance precisely so they could practice such invasive medicine, getting right to the heart of things.

. . .

Med school has a way of making metaphors literal. When you say you have touched someone's heart, sometimes you have. And sometimes it becomes clear that the literal and metaphorical are closely tied.

Mackenzie touched a literal heart that night, but it also touched her metaphorical heart. As the case wound down to the patient's demise, Mackenzie's feelings surged.

"I didn't want him to be alone. We were all there, but he was still sort of alone. So, I was trying to rub his leg a little bit, which is silly maybe." The fellow asked her if she was okay, and she responded, "Yeah, it's just that he's not okay."

Mackenzie wanted to comfort a dying man. Doing so in that moment marked her out from the surgeons. The surgeons preferred humor as a coping mechanism, teasing each other about the body's shapes, smells, and sounds. When they teased students to watch their shoes for leaking fluids, they were testing the students. Tease back and you belong. It wasn't Mackenzie's way. She felt that the surgeons had remarkable bedside manners and technical skills, but she wondered where they kept their emotions when working through multiple traumas every call night.

"I think there must be some level of suppression because seeing that four times a night all the time seems like . . . I don't know. I think that's not a strength that I have. I have other strengths, but that is not one of them."

Thinking ahead to her Match, Mackenzie wants to be a primary care physician. She has settled on the choice between two varieties of primary care: family medicine or internal medicine. Surgery confirmed that for her.

If she encounters a patient who is wheezing, she wants to think about not only the physiology of wheezing but also the pollution that increases wheezing. She wants to know everything about the people she meets as patients. For her, the hardest part of surgery was delimiting her interest to a single problem.

She admires the surgeons and learns from their teaching, but they are not the people with whom she will cast her lot. She will become a primary care physician. "Something about behavior change in general is something that really interests me. I think it goes with addiction and other chronic disease management things. It requires setting goals, being able to make incremental change over time, and developing perseverance against something that is very overwhelming and challenging for people." She might do a fellowship in addiction medicine as well. "It's something that is very needed, and I like the idea of being able to contribute to that. There were a couple of times on internal medicine when there was time for me to stay and listen to folks who struggled with addiction. There's a lot of trauma there, and a lot of listening required. I think sometimes people just want to be heard."

And that is where the downward arrow took Mackenzie. She found the core belief that will hold her captive for the rest of her life: *I listen to people to help so they can make changes they cannot make on their own.* She learned about the three Ds (depression, divorce, and drink)— the shorthand for the many internal dangers threatening a physician's well-being—while she confronted the final *D* (death). Despite all the emotional risks of listening to the ill as a primary care physician, Mackenzie is still placing her bet on being that kind of listener.

Chapter 12

HANG-UPS

*M*ALLORY MYERS AND MAGGIE KRIZ walk past a patient, just a few years older than the two of them, who is mumbling to herself about all the things no one else knows. They can make out that the patient is saying that her father is the president, but she is the one who invented cellphones, so she is the one who deserves untold riches. They can hear her muttering about how she is the one whose life was ruined by vampire hypnotists. They can see her black T-shirt and its message: in block pink letters, "REALITY CALLED," and underneath, in white script, *"And I hung up."*

Mallory and Maggie are visiting the hospital's adult inpatient psychiatric ward to learn how a physician can listen so well that she learns what even patients do not know about themselves. Mallory and Maggie are two of several learners on that day's psychiatry team. A pair of medical students in the traditional clinical year are rotating on the service for an entire month. The traditional med students spend their first half day getting oriented—a tour of the unit, a tour of the EHR, a tour of the bathrooms and fire extinguishers—before seeing patients. LIC students like Mallory and Maggie skip the half-day tour; they are already familiar with the hospital and with many of the patients they will see.

Maggie joined rounds so she could visit a middle-aged woman whom she follows with Dr. Stichman as an outpatient. Stichman does not see patients on the psych ward, but Maggie can. The woman attempted suicide and was still ambivalent about her survival. Many students try to swap a patient's ambivalence for a clinician's confidence: *You are lucky to be alive. You can be treated. You can do well. You take meds. You go to therapy. You get better.* They slather these well-meant assertions on like an emotional topcoat.

Maggie has a deeper confidence. She knows the patient, and they both know that this is just one day they will have together. She does not need to ask the demographic questions—name, age, gender, insurance, emergency contact, allergies, and the like—that dominate initial medical encounters. She does not have to wrap the encounter up in an artificial way. She sits with a sufferer whom she is starting to know well. Gradually, the woman meets Maggie's eyes and promises to see her again.

Ambivalence bested by continuity; Hirsh and Ogur would be proud.

. . .

Psych wards are good places to learn how to listen like a doctor. Many students, including Catherine Ard, worked on a psych ward before medical school. Psych wards are chronically understaffed, so they often hire people who are more eager than experienced. For the people who can navigate safely through the psych ward, it can add essential skills for future physicians. But safety is never promised. Working on a psych unit is one of the most dangerous work environments in the country; while the average hospital worker is six times more likely to be intentionally injured at work than the average American worker, the average psychiatric hospital worker is fifty-nine times more likely [75]. By finding her way through the ward, Catherine realized that she had been preparing to become a physician all along.

When she graduated from college, medical school was an abandoned childhood dream. Catherine tried out other futures. She nannied a bit. She worked in a hot dog stand, a cheese store, a pie shop, and a bar. It all left her wanting something more. She joined Teach for America. They assigned her to a middle school in a Texas border town. She would rise at 4:00 or 5:00 a.m. so she could be at the school by 6:00 a.m. When she arrived, she pushed a cart around the school, joining whichever class needed a teacher. She would abruptly enter a vacant educational space and bring order to a disorderly classroom. She learned how hard you must work to survive as a teacher.

"I didn't realize going into teaching, how much of it was going to be physical performing, you're performing all day long. I remember other teachers saying in the beginning, 'Don't let them see you smile until January.' I tried. I tried to be that kind of teacher, but that style was never going to work for me. I think kids could feel I was faking it."

Catherine did not want to fake it. She did not want to float in and out of other people's lives. She wanted fuller relationships or none at all. "I love those relationships that I built with some of my students, and in those brief moments, I saw some things that I wanted to try to re-create in a future career." Some things, but not enough. Teaching exhausted her. "I got pretty burnt out in those couple of years. I thought, 'Maybe people who are just doing a desk job thing have the right idea. They're working their nine to five, and then going home and doing something after that.'"

She moved back to Colorado and worked in the correspondence office of a retirement company. It was more predictable than teaching but less meaningful. "After a little while, even just working a 40-hour week there felt so much longer than working a 60- or an 80-hour week doing something that I cared about. I was bored. There were some good people there, but I wasn't surrounded by the type of people that I really wanted to be surrounded by."

Then a fluke injury changed her surroundings. Shuttling between doctor's visits and physical therapy appointments to repair a torn ACL, Catherine's childhood dream resurfaced. To figure out if she could realize her doctor dreams, she signed up for the prerequisite courses Flexner mandated for medical school admission at a local community college. At the same time, she traded her comfortable desk job for an uncomfortable health care gig. Behavioral health techs walk the floor on inpatient psych units to check on patients, breaking up fights, talking people down, and running clinical errands. The work is as hard as teaching, but with adults experiencing some of the worst days of their life instead of children learning on one of their ordinary days. Catherine gravitated to the hardest unit, the ward for adults experiencing psychosis. She learned to listen to people who had hung up on reality. She connected with people whom others could not reach.

"We didn't have any kind of security or anything there. It was all just us. The person I worked with the most, he and I really relied on our relationships with the patients and our verbal de-escalation skills. We had a similar philosophy of, 'Hey, if we respect these people, they'll probably respect us.' Most of the time, that worked."

It was like teaching. Some people assumed the worst. Don't smile until January. Catherine and her coworker assumed the best. Smile daily. "When I was working my shift with my coworker, he and I had very similar vibes and very similar approaches to patients. When I worked other shifts with other people who were more aggressive, and probably a little more defensive, it was totally different. It was like the teaching environment where people were like, 'Oh, you really have to be a hard ass and be disciplined to get these people in line.' And my approach was always like, 'No, I just have to show them that I care about them.' And, you know, that approach works for me, and maybe it doesn't work for you. But in both of those environments, I found that the more that I kind of dug in and just showed people that I was going to treat them with respect and that I cared about them, the better things went."

. . .

In the week's Thursday class, the LIC students are learning an aspect of this lesson from Professor Jackie Glover, a philosopher who visits to teach about how to ask permission like a professional. It's one of the first steps in treating a person with respect: seek consent.

Glover defines informed consent, the process by which a clinician explains and receives permission to perform (or not perform) a clinical act, and then asks students to discuss what informed consent really looks like. Itzam Marin says, "In the preclinical years, informed consent seemed black and white. In the clinical year, with real medicine, it all seems gray." Sarah Bardwell observes that she witnessed informed consent, but it never feels like a real choice. "Our job is to save people, to cure people. But maybe they no longer want a cure. We always seem to come in with our opinions. And we say, 'this might be an outcome,' but might is an underestimation. 'Might' often means waking up with a colostomy." Sarah has seen patients awaken to a post-operative reality, like bodily waste accumulating in a bag attached to the skin, radically different from the one to which they consented.

Megan Kalata chimes in. "I feel like there is ideally and realistically. Ideally, it's checking to make sure you're not imposing on someone. It's giving them a checklist with options. Realistically, it's a legal discussion. It's saying that I told someone so they can't sue me."

Maggie adds, "There's a difference between explaining and telling. I felt like so many of the conversations used ambiguous terms to cover lots of stuff. 'You have a risk of infection.' But when you think about health literacy, it's never a true explanation."

Glover explains that a thorough informed consent includes a diagnosis, a proposed clinical action, a discussion of the action's risks and benefits, alternative clinical actions, and the risk and benefits of declining treatment. "Have you witnessed anyone conduct a thorough informed consent?"

One or two students nod. Most have not. Glover surfaces the unspoken expectation that patients, especially poor patients, ought to or must accept a physician's counsel as a price of receiving care. Glover introduces the concept of capacity, the ability of a patient to make decisions for herself. Capacity can change with a patient's condition.

Maggie volunteers that she saw patients whose care was deferred until capacity was regained and consent was possible. "I remember the first time I was on the surgical trauma service. I would walk around and there would be people sitting in the halls. I realized that they were intoxicated, and the team was waiting for them to come down so that they had capacity to consent for treatment. They needed surgical drainage of abscesses from skin popping. They needed to sober up so they could be intubated, but it seemed unethical for them to be withdrawing in the hallway."

Several students nod; they have also watched patients stay in the emergency department until they have completed withdrawal from opiates or alcohol before they could receive definitive treatment.

Picking up the theme, Sarah says, "It feels to me like someone has capacity if they agree with the team, and they don't have capacity if they disagree with the team."

The students laugh darkly and nod.

Mallory adds, "I saw this new patient. He lived alone. He had diabetes and they needed to amputate his leg. He agreed. But I wondered if he understood what that meant. I asked my preceptor, and they said it was okay."

Sarah responds, "It feels sometimes like instead of explaining a situation to a patient, physicians just say the same thing over and over."

Mackenzie Garcia agrees: "And then the patient just repeats it back to them! Yes, that happens so often."

The students discuss the many instances in which patients decline interpreters. Mackenzie says, "I have times when a woman declines her interpreter, and her husband speaks for her. I can understand him and know he is not translating but summarizing."

Summarizing instead of translating—this is the kind of difference Glover wants students to see. When a physician simply summarizes what could happen, good or bad, in a medical encounter, it is not a true consent. Glover wants the students to think of a true consent as more like translating the language of medicine into language a patient truly speaks, so they can make their best decision. A true consent reduces the imbalance of power between physician and patient, bridging the gap between those who know the body and those who know the community.

Glover says, "It doesn't feel good to just do things *to* someone, it feels good to do things *for* someone. If you just wanted to do things to someone, you would go to veterinary school." Glover is getting students to see the differences between being a physician and other kinds of professionals. A physician engages in acts—dissecting bodies, performing intimate examinations, asking after dark secrets, prescribing mind- and body-altering medications—that are assaultive outside the physician-patient relationship. Being a good physician means being a good person, the kind who explains a treatment, the kind who serves someone else. Maggie concludes, "Thinking about informed consent shows me how powerful this job is."

. . .

On the psych ward, Catherine saw the difference that treating people with care and respect made. "We had really great relationships with our patients, even patients that had histories of violence. I remember one guy was scary when he first came in, but we worked hard to try to talk to him and show him respect. And there was something in his room that maintenance needed to fix. So, they went in there, they fixed

it, they left and then he walks in his room, and he just started screaming, 'Hey, hey, hey, something's wrong!' And we go in there and they
had left a razor blade in his room. He's just pointing to it. 'That's not
mine. I didn't bring it in here. They left it. Please take it and get it out of
here.' I like having that relationship with people, where we could make
it a very trusting place to be."

She trusted, and it proved trustworthy. She applied to medical
school. The school placed her on the waitlist. She thought that medical school would be another year away, so she committed to another
psych tech job out of state, and then the call came in. Someone left med
school because of a family emergency—as luck would have it, another
woman named Catherine, as if med students were actors with
understudies—during the first week, and the dean of admissions was
offering acceptance to her, if she could start immediately. "It felt a little
bit like divine intervention, so I drove back, full of energy, and started
up that week." Early in med school, Catherine met Dr. Adams and
heard her talk about the LIC. It reminded her of the best parts of all the
jobs she had held before.

"Coming into medicine, I had this vague idea of wanting to try to
help and make the world a better place, but I didn't really have a picture
of what that would look like. And so, Denver Health kind of immediately gave me a picture of what that could look like."

. . .

Three times a year, Adams asks her future physicians to reflect on what
medicine is looking like for each of them. Adams tells the students to
take a break from the rote clinical writing—progress notes, procedure
notes, and sign-out notes—that summarizes encounters. Adams asks
students to write reflectively, describing not what occurred in a clinical encounter but how it feels and what it means. Adams prompts students to write on how poverty affects access to care, on the boundaries
between patients and practitioners, and on terminating relationships

with patients. For each essay, faculty provide written feedback. Over the years, Adams has observed that students most often reflect on what it means to be altruistic when caring for the underserved, how to build therapeutic alliances, how to practice humility and gratitude, how to be resilient through difficult encounters, and what they aspire to be as physicians [76].

Early in the year, Maggie wrote that she was told that the LIC would allow her to provide more real care for the patients than anyone else on the team, but she realized what they meant only during her internal medicine immersion: "We have more time to talk with people—sit with them and give them a shoulder to cry on, a hand to hold, or just a person to tell their story to and truly feel heard. One of the most powerful antidotes to any ailment: listening." Like Catherine before her, Maggie was learning how to listen like a doctor.

"Doctors have a very peculiar job—it is their profession to sit with patients and their families through the best and worst moments of their lives," Maggie found. "It is an incredible honor to be present for strangers—to be a friendly face, a trusted confidant, a patient teacher." But she observed that this is not a one-way process: "In helping people you open yourself up—make yourself vulnerable to the pain and joy your patients feel. This year I have seen patients make a complete recovery from life-threatening vasculitis, give birth to healthy twin boys, repeatedly fall into psychosis and mania, quit injecting heroin, get adopted out of foster care, and die with their families at their side. In allowing me to be a part of their lives, all the patients I have worked with have left an imprint that has shaped what kind of doctor I will become."

The reflective writing helps students like Maggie process who and what they are becoming. Adams hopes it will preserve their initial empathy, while focusing it into a physician's social empathy, the ability to imagine the lived experience of others [77].

That is part of the work of becoming companions with the ill. And to prove that it is working, Adams asked a former LIC student, Dr. Robbie Flick, to interview thirty patients who were seen at least three times by an LIC student. Flick found that when the patients spoke about the LIC students, they talked about the students as being on their side.

She made me feel good.

He visited me.

She asked about my kids.

He knew me.

They understood.

I could tell her anything.

He was a comfort to me.

When they were there, I felt like we could do this together.

The relationships with students sustained the patients even when the systems of society—schools, hospitals, churches, governments—failed them [78]. Flick's work suggested that the program was more mutual than most medical training models—benefiting the patients and students alike. So Adams kept studying. She interviewed more of her students, as well as LIC students from other schools in Ireland and Scotland. Adams found that the LIC was more than the continuity celebrated by Hirsh and Ogur. The LIC created relationships where students could connect with patients, even when reality called, and become true companions of the ill [79].

Adams needs research findings like this to keep growing the LIC. She is working toward a future where it becomes the model for all of medicine, while simultaneously training this year's students to listen so well that they can form the sustaining relationships that previous students, like Catherine, have already developed.

. . .

Mallory is learning, even when she meets new patients. Back on the psych ward, none of Mallory's patients are hospitalized on this day, so she accompanies a psychiatry resident to see a patient newly admitted to the unit, a clean but institutional space. There are no doorknobs on the doors or hooks on the wall, since those count as ligature risks. The hand sanitizer dispensers are often disabled because patients with an alcohol use disorder have been found crouching underneath their motion sensors, triggering them again and again so that they can drink their measured doses for their scant alcohol content. No matter what country songs say, hand sanitizer shots on the psych unit are the most desperate of drinks. And the furniture in this kind of watering hole is weighted to prevent it from being picked up and thrown. The space is designed for safety, but the effect is to compel change. It is architecture arrayed against ambivalence [75].

Mallory finds a seat in one of the unit's secure chairs, alongside the resident. The resident starts off by getting the demographics from Malik (middle-aged man, HIV+, history of depression, maybe bipolar) and the reason for hospitalization (suicidal thoughts and a plan to slice his wrists). She efficiently presses for the details. Malik is a telemarketer by day but homeless by night. He sought shelter from a community agency, but they told him he could not receive their support without his HIV meds. They referred Malik to the hospital to restart his meds, and during that evaluation he divulged thoughts of suicide. The resident speeds through the rest of the history of present illness and the review of systems, asking the pressing questions like a harried physician, and then abruptly stops and looks to Mallory.

Mallory leans forward, off the back of the chair and into her opportunity. Her tone is engaged but calm. Her questions are neutral but thorough. She can elicit what the resident could not: an emotion. Malik cries. He talks about his mother, who had struggled with depression. He talks about his maternal grandmother, who had suicided with rat poison. Mallory listens, never panicking, never betraying fear. She asks directly about his suicide attempt and the blood it produced, all her past squeamishness about blood erased by the power of serving someone in need. "Tell me about being suicidal. Were you ever suicidal before?"

Malik reports a similar period of depression with suicidal thoughts seventeen years ago.

Mallory nods. "What is different about this time?"

"Back then, I had a job. I had a future. I had a lady in my life. Now, I have nothing. Emotionally, I don't care anymore. Then, I had people in my life. Now, I have no people in my life."

Mallory listens, hearing how the patient lost his community, and then listens some more. The reflective writing sessions, the Thursday afternoon teachings, the advice of students who went before her—it all helps Mallory access her own emotions. Mallory has experienced depression as well. She signed up for the LIC to have a consistent team of classmates and teachers, as well as patients—people in her life. It is still hard. Burnout shadows her steps, but she hopes to someday flourish as a physician because the work gives her a sense of purpose. She silently relates not only to times in your life when you do not care anymore but also to the benefits of having people in your life. She stays in the physician's role. She does not burden Malik with her own experiences. She does not hang up on her emotions. She uses them to listen. The resident has more medical knowledge, but Mallory hears more. She learns Malik better because she elicits his emotions while accessing her own emotions, like a physician.

Chapter 13

MANIFESTED CHECKLISTS

SARAH BARDWELL KEEPS checklists—what to do each day, how the doing changes her, what items she needs to survive the changes. Working through the lists brings her dreams to life. Manifesting checklists has become one of her coping mechanisms. The checklists keep Sarah on task.

On surgery, she rises at a monkish 3:30 a.m. to start the list. On other services, she sleeps in until a farmer's 5:00 a.m. Either way, the list is long enough to shorten the time for breakfast. Most mornings, she runs on coffee until about noon. "I don't even eat food at tables anymore. Most of the time, it's over a computer. I put a lot of consideration into what foods I can eat with one hand."

Sarah makes other considerations for food prep at this point in the clinical year: no vegetables, no cooking. Vegetables spoil. Cooking takes time.

"I was really pretty good for the first year and half of med school. I did a lot of crockpot cooking. But I don't cook for myself anymore. Even the amount of time that it takes to think of ingredients, go to the store and get them, cut them into pieces, and put them in a crockpot is . . ." She shakes her head from side to side, like a disapproving parent.

"Sometimes I wonder, 'Could I make time?' But then I realize, 'Oh, no,' from start to finish that effort is maybe an hour long. I live very close to a grocery store that I never go to."

The time isn't the only reason she can't bring herself to cook: the energy she has for keeping up with her list has dimmed as the year has gone on. She can now complete only its absolute essentials. And her idea of what counts as essential has changed.

"I stopped brushing my teeth at night. I do brush my teeth in the morning. I've stopped flossing too. It's just 30 seconds, but I can't handle it. I don't know. I used to plan my diet around the idea of eating seven servings of fruits and vegetables every day and high-protein meals. And I used to do physical therapy every night, just stretches and things. I used to go to the gym."

While friends still make the essentials list, Sarah expects them to take the initiative. "My friends are pretty good about being like, 'Hi. I haven't seen you in two months.' And we'll get a coffee some morning or something."

Sarah also keeps a list of all she gives up so she can, someday, reclaim it. "I have a sticky note by my bed of all of the healthy habits that I hope to one day readopt into my life."

In the meantime, Sarah makes notes of where to find food adjacent to (or even within) clinical settings. Students like Sarah quickly learn which hospital services have morning bagels and afternoon lunches and which nurses allow students to share in the overnight potlucks they host in the break rooms. Students learn which meals are worth eating in the hospital's basement cafeteria; which supply closets store individual servings of graham crackers and peanut butter that, when freed from their plastic wrapping, can quickly lift low blood sugar; and which ICUs deliver Cheerios to the bedsides of the comatose patients who can never eat them. Students bring food for each other on Thursday afternoons because they know how hard it is to eat well, and they advise each other to put "eat breakfast" on their to-do lists so that at least one required activity will be personally pleasurable.

On other days, students eat in the crevices of time between activities. Sarah likes to bicycle, but never on Tuesdays, which she splits between a morning session on the eastern edge of Denver and an afternoon session downtown.

"I have to be back on this campus within an hour. But I never really leave at noon, and I have to eat lunch, and it would just be too hard to ride my bike and eat lunch at the same time, but I can drive and eat lunch at the same time."

The moral: never drive closely behind a med student.

Sarah is a master list maker, but there's one list no medical student can avoid being chained to: the one they must open on their computer every time they encounter a person as a patient. Admitting a patient? Peck out a history and physical. Following up with a patient? Update a progress note. Sending a patient home? Check your way through the boxes on a discharge summary.

The computer provides prompts. When an admission note is opened, a physical exam autopopulates, prompting the student to chart a physical exam from head to toe:

> Head: atraumatic, PERRLA, EOMI, no murmurs/masses/
> bruits, thyroid at midline. *Click.*
> Chest: RRR, NL S1/S2, lungs CTA bil. *Click.*
> Abdomen: soft, NT/ND, BS*4. *Click.*
> GU: deferred. *Click.*
> Extremities: no C/C/E. *Click.*
> Neuro: CN II–XII intact, WNL. *Click.*

The inscrutable abbreviations are for initiates, but even an inexperienced student can click through them all in a matter of seconds.

Someone with more experience knows what each acronym and abbreviation stands for, the signs of bodily organs in health and sickness, designed to tell other clinicians about the patient's condition. Or at least that is what they used to stand for. Once, WNL meant *Within Normal Limits*, that the physical exam findings fell within the expected range of normal. Physicians now joke that it means *We Never Looked*, only clicking the box to make sure the documentation is complete for the administrators, regulators, and insurers who are its true audience today. When a student makes a list and checks things off it, it does not necessarily correspond to the reality of something happening for a patient.

The late physician-writer Oliver Sacks observed that every era demands and rewards different skills of physicians. Sacks remembers that one of his physician father's leading clinical skills was his sense of smell: "my father had an acute sense of smell as a young man, and like all doctors of his generation, he depended on it when seeing patients. He could detect the smell of diabetic urine or of a putrid lung abscess as soon as he entered a person's house" [80, p. 46]. Physicians diagnosed disease and charted treatment progress with their sense of smell.

Sarah and her colleagues are rarely asked to use their sense of smell to diagnose. When asked directly, they can recall hospital smells with antiseptic top notes and undernotes of something organic and unclean, but they do not connect smells to diagnoses like pater Sacks.

Maggie Kriz was surprised by how little she smelled, even when a patient's body was open before her in the operating room. She had worked at a homeless shelter; she knew how smells indicated particular deprivations and diseases. The operating room smelled, well, less.

"You walk in, and it has this sort of strange smell. It's almost weird. It's a hard smell to describe because it's like a lack of smell, just total lack of smell." She could smell cleaning supplies and a weird stale smell but not the patient.

"We had one patient who bled out seven liters. We had to call a mass transfusion protocol, and it was just strange." The patient was nearing death, but the anesthesia made him appear as if he was simply sleeping, and his smell offered few clues of his condition. It is what Maggie could see that explained the patient's health.

"It's more intimate and less intimate at the same time, because you're literally cutting someone open and seeing their body in a way that no one has seen before and seeing their anatomy and being able to see the choices that they've made in their liver or their lungs, but you're not talking to them." Maggie paused. "I expected to be able to smell the blood and stuff and you just really can't. Even when we had that mass transfusion and there was so much blood."

The students do not live in an era of diagnostic smells; they could be successful even if they developed anosmia and completely lost their sense of smell. The students live in an era of documentation in the EHR; they could never be successful if they developed agraphia and lost their ability to document. This era's clinical adage: *if an event is not documented, it never occurred.*

Documentation is the way a clinician organizes her thinking. Documentation is the way care teams speak to each other across their disciplinary divisions. Documentation is the way a clinician translates her time into money. Documentation is the way auditors assess compliance with regulations. Documentation is the way lawyers assess whether the standards of care have been met. Smelling is a diagnostic tool; documenting in the EHR is the very system of contemporary care. If the EHR goes offline in a contemporary hospital, clinical services sputter to a stop.

Documentation serves so many needs. Hence, clinicians serve the needs of documentation. Today, for every hour physicians spend seeing patients, they spend almost two additional hours documenting in the electronic record. At the workday's end, most physicians have not completed their documentation, so physicians typically spend an additional hour or two each worknight, as Dr. Boyle warned, documenting [81]. Students learn that today's physicians spend more time with EHRs than with patients.

Students learn that many physicians carry headphones to use while sitting at workstations to code in the EHR. Hospitals replace private physician offices with open cubicles. The offices were decorated with books and diplomas and photos. The cubicles are decorated with tip sheets and documentation guides and the number for IT support. Many could be cleaned out in less time than it would take to write another progress note. The workrooms look like call centers, everyone bunkered down, documenting, and eating one-handed lunches while gazing into the computer. The smells are beside the point.

The longer the list at the hospital got for Sarah, the longer her list of the ways in which she is personally being sickened. Medical training is affecting her spirit, her body, and her sleep.

"I've pretty much adapted to sleeping five and a half hours at night. I didn't ever think it would be possible. I used to sleep thirteen hours a night. I was in the best health of my life before I started medical school."

She feels her body being degraded by the work. She feels the decade age difference from her classmates. She spent her own twenties running her health down, before returning to college so she could learn about health. In the years leading up to med school, she slept, ate, and exercised well. She lifted weights, danced, and hiked her way back to health while simultaneously realizing she could learn math and science. She felt like she was growing.

"School, up until med school, was great. I had a great time. I was learning for the first time."

Medical school felt like a regression. She feels less like a learner and more like a follower of instructions. As she checks items off medicine's list, her own list is left undone.

Though coming to medical school later in life has certain advantages—added perspective, sometimes added motivation—Sarah feels the drawbacks. "I'm tired. My mind is not very fast. I have to work really hard to learn things. I believe that there are a lot of people in their twenties who also have to work, but I notice the difference. I'm fatigued." When other students moan about studying until 4:00 a.m., she is incredulous. "I can work until 4:00, but I cannot study medicine until 4:00 in the morning. I have to tap out by 11:00 p.m. That's the point at which I can no longer, with any utility, put information in my mind."

She worries about osteoporosis—it runs in her family—every time her back hurts and thinks about how she has lost bone mass and gained weight. "I'm in the last haul of being able to create bone mass. And I'm not going to." She feels the loss of control of both her body and her time. She wonders why all the learning during the clinical year must come at a personal cost. Several friends have fallen away. "By the time I get out of this, I don't even know who's going to be around that will even talk to me anymore." Luckily, her family is still supportive. She feels like they are truly impressed with her efforts, even proud of her, for what feels like the first time.

Romantically, there have been ups and downs. She literally lacked time for her husband in medical school. Getting divorced is on her checklist, but they will finalize the separation only, she says, "whenever he gets around to that." She cannot muster the time or energy to pursue it herself. In the meantime, she has a new boyfriend who supports her work. "He does my laundry for me, and he cooks for me. He brings me food in bowls, just short of spoon-feeding me."

She can eat soup with one hand, hunched over a computer, so the other hand can document and keep the list that keeps her.

. . .

A few weeks later, Sarah explains what makes her lists worth keeping.

"We had a patient with rectal cancer. We were sitting there in pre-op explaining the risks of the procedure and the risk that he will have an ostomy, the risk that he will have a permanent ostomy, and the risk that he would have a total rectal resection and an ostomy for the rest of his life. And the patient says that he really hopes that he doesn't have a permanent ostomy because he's a religious man. And the surgeon's like, 'Here, sign this.' And then we moved on.

"And I thought a lot about that. I wondered, 'Why would it be important if he was a religious man?' And then during the surgery, they ended up taking everything out. He had no anus, no rectum, he would forever have an ostomy, and it looked like he might have a permanent urinary catheter. I went to talk with him afterward, and it occurred to me that the reason why it was important that he's religious is because he can't kill himself. And so, if he ended up on the other side of this surgery with a life that he does not want to live, he would be stuck in that."

She sighed, "We don't explain ourselves very well." What vexed Sarah most was that she often saw this in medicine, partly due to different perceptions of risk. When surgeons said that there is a risk of an ostomy, they were thinking, "We do ostomies all the time. It's not a big deal to us if you have an ostomy. Physiologically speaking, you're going to be fine." But, as she wryly observes, "None of those surgeons have ostomies." Living for a time, or the rest of your life, with a surgical opening in your abdomen where bodily waste collects is the kind of life-altering event that makes the power of medicine almost too real.

"It occurred to me that there is a really broad gap in perspectives that the patient and the surgeon have in terms of what it means to be okay at the end of the surgery. And we don't do a very good job of really making sure that people understand what it really means to do whatever it is that we're doing.

"That was a life-changing experience. I spent a long time talking with that guy about how he didn't want to be alive because of something that we did to him."

She also feels what the hospital is doing to her. She loves the LIC but is starting to doubt the utility of medical school. Yet she still works toward her goal, to effect some amount of positive change in the world and for people in her community. The problem, she is realizing, is that medicine might not be the best way to achieve social change. Or, even if it's possible to effect change, she fears that, by the end of training, "I'm not going to have the energy to even try."

. . .

Sarah rests her remaining hopes on matching in family medicine. She likes that the pace of family medicine is slower, the changes incremental. Slow medicine acknowledging that only some things can get done today, that care can be a continual process, that a physician and patient can bend habits toward health. "For some people, the idea of working with a patient on quitting smoking or losing weight over five years is totally miserable, pull-your-hair-off frustration. To me, it's a perfectly fine pace. I have no problem with that." She acknowledges that, even in this specialty, "you never get a chance to address everybody's problems, and everybody's a little frustrated because of that. But you get to know people, you hear their stories. I at least get to listen to all of their problems, even if I don't have time to address all of their problems."

She reflected on a particular patient she met in the family medicine clinic and then followed through surgery and post-op. The patient, a young mother who had immigrated to America, potentially had Lynch syndrome, which puts patients at a higher risk for many types of cancer. Sarah acknowledged the many medical procedures facing the patient, like any medical student, but was especially grateful for the opportunity to meet the patient's family and pastor. Sarah had an opportunity to understand the context of her patient's life. Sarah got to know her well enough that she could pick up on the range of emotions and fears she was experiencing: she knew that when she was very quiet in pre-op, it was because she was scared. Then, after the surgery, Sarah attuned to her pain. This was hard, but the hard that Sarah wanted: to be persistently present, not just click through a checklist.

As Sarah ranged through her own emotions and experiences, as she learned to eat with one hand and tend to the EHR with the other, she held on to shards of gratitude. She was no longer sure about medical school or medicine, but she still loves Denver Health. She still loves the LIC's flexibility. She still loves following patients across the system. She still loves persistently being present. And so she keeps a good list.

Sarah even keeps a list of the things that she carries so she can make it through the clinical year: cram-books and clinical algorithms, a penlight and stethoscope, lip balm and sunscreen, lotion and deodorant, antidepressant and antihistamines, spoons and forks, and other expected things. Then, she adds that she carries "the hopes of all my friends and family, the guilt of my father's help and money, the burden of my loans, the damp leaden fear of failure in every moment, heavy eyelids, usually an insulated lunch bag with two to three meals—almost always a fruit and yogurt smoothie, turkey sandwich with apple and snap peas, and 2 cups of chicken and veggie soup—deep preoccupation for my patients who have missed their appointments but whose voice-mails are always full, an abundance of tears that can be conjured at nearly any moment, a heart soggy with the sadness and fear of those facing illness and death, a love of palliative care medicine, a love of family medicine, a well of brightly effervescent admiration for the strength and will of so many people who graciously allow me to witness their lives, a deeply humbling gratitude for my teachers in all their forms."

She hopes her list will carry her through.

Chapter 14

KILLING YOUR NUMBER

*T*HE FIVE *F*s are the differential for a distended abdomen: Fat, Fluid, Flatus, Feces, and Fetus."

"I didn't even know that a gallbladder had an ejection fraction."

"That's it—the X-ray shows a cobra in the chest!"

Dr. Vishnu Kulasekaran is leading a chalice exercise, an hourlong case on SOB—shortness of breath—in adults. Working through the case, the students develop a physician's response—differential diagnosis, assessment, and treatment plan—while speaking their version of doctor talk.

Kulasekaran sits at the front of the room, laughing along with the nerdy mnemonics and the bad jokes and then gently nudging them back into the case, where he invites students to interpret X-rays for disease processes rather than exotic animals.

Mallory Myers starts. "The airway is patent as far as we can tell. I can only count eight ribs. The cardiac silhouette looks normal, not enlarged. There's something funky going on in the upper right—I think they are calcifications. The diaphragm looks flattened. It looks like COPD."

Kulasekaran nods. Itzam Marin interprets pulmonary function test results. "It has a pattern of obstructive lung disease pretty consistent with COPD." Chronic obstructive pulmonary disease it is;

now he needs the kind of details a physician builds a treatment plan around.

As Kulasekaran's attention moves around the room, one student interprets the labs: "Respiratory acidosis has induced a metabolic alkalosis." Then another student explains the treatment: "We ordered prednisone, but we went back and forth on azithromycin."

Maggie Kriz concludes, "We think he is having a COPD exacerbation. Increased SOB, wheezing, sputum, and cough."

Kulasekaran qualifies: "Based on the guidelines, he's on the fence. I don't think you'd be wrong in following him or empirically treating him. And where do you want to treat him? That's the other decision point you're at. Should he be treated in the clinic and head home, or would you send him to the hospital?"

The students start riffing. They change parts of the clinical story—symptoms, age, gender—and assess how each changes the case. Treatments change, outcomes shift, but the students never speak of how much each change costs or who will pay those costs. Like the faculty, med students rarely talk openly about how much being a doctor will pay or how much it will cost their patients. It's the variable in every case about which they say they least.

· · ·

Except Sarah Bardwell.

She worked for a decade more than the other students before even contemplating her career switch. When she decided on medicine, she looked up the starting wage of a family physician at the place she planned to practice—Denver Health—and was initially heartened by her back-of-the-envelope calculation. "It was $180 grand. So take-home after taxes, $120,000. After taxes, you know, that's a pretty big chunk of money."

She is now no longer sure that, at least from a financial sense, she will come out ahead.

"If you break it down—which I have done, and it's a horrifying thing for me, so I talk about it all the time—if you take $120,000 and you work an eighty-hour week, you make $35 an hour. Which is not peanuts, but it's significantly less than I could make bartending—and it's hard work. I didn't come into this for the money at all." Bardwell shakes her head, "The more I started thinking about the paycheck, the more attached I've become to it."

The paychecks are still in the future. Unlike bartending, medicine requires a decade of expensive training.

"So, 35 bucks an hour, I'm kind of like, 'Whoa, that's bad. That's terrible. If I had known . . .'" Her voice trails off while she thinks of her own number. Then she finds her resolve again.

"Whatever. It wouldn't have made a difference for me because I'm not here for the money. But I would have thought twice."

As Sarah counts time and money, she also factors in opportunity costs: all the living she is forgoing to become a physician. She entered medicine because she wanted to care for people, but some days the calculation does not add up.

. . .

Med students often run the numbers over and over in their minds, during idle moments in the library and lecture hall, even in the clinic and the ward.

They calculate time. Assuming no delays, med school is four years. Then there are three more years of residency if you become a primary care physician, up to ten years if you want to be a subspecialist. Assuming no missteps, you will be a newly minted physician in— minimum—seven years, the better part of a decade. A decade where any income will be exceeded by many expenses: application fees, tuition payments, rent checks, and grocery bills.

They count money. The median annual cost of medical school is $39,149 for in-state students at a public school and $62,948 at a private school [82]. With interest, a medical student can easily be out $300K for tuition alone before she begins residency, during which she will earn a $60K salary for caring for the sick for up to eighty hours a week. Assuming eighty hours for forty-eight weeks a year, this comes to $15.63 an hour, before taxes.

Sometimes, when bored and bitter on rounds or in lecture, students will calculate how much a wasted hour or ineffectual lecture is costing them. It is expensive, in time and money, to be known as a physician. Many students fantasize often of their numbers, the years that will pass and the dollars they will pay, to reach the moment when all their debts are paid.

The students are not alone in this fantasy. Many of the patients at Denver Health have spent time in the correctional system. They talk about "killing your number," completing the number of days, months, or years in which you are awaiting trial, serving time in a correctional facility, or finishing out probation.

When a student's calculations of time and money govern their thoughts, obscuring reminders of why they pursued medicine, they are killing their number too. On bad days, they become embittered, wondering why someone had not explained the costs better. They had received only brief lectures on finances at the beginning and end of med school, but these were more about the mechanics of student loans than about how money affects the way you practice medicine and the kind of person you become.

Any rational review concludes that money distorts the practice of medicine and the lives of physicians. America spends twice as much on health care, per capita, than other high-income countries but has the lowest life expectancy and the highest suicide rate [83]. America also produces fewer nurses and physicians than most developing countries, so it is not the training of professionals that makes our care so expensive; it is the cost of those services. America spends literally twice as much, per capita, as our neighbors to the north in Canada [84], and one in every four dollars Americans spend on health care is wasted [85].

And even more than the thorough financial counseling students sometimes wish they had received in training, what physicians are missing about the flow of money in medicine is how a physician's choices alter the finances of their patients.

Students are tasked with learning to diagnose and treat, even how to reduce waste, but are offered only general training on how much their care will cost. They are taught the differences between different forms of health insurance, but explaining how much each test, medicine, and treatment will cost each patient is so complex and varied that it is not taught. Fewer still learn how the trillion-dollar health care industry distorts the relationships between physicians; the students can feel it anyway.

. . .

When Sarah was considering medicine, she called physicians and asked to shadow them, so she could test her own dream. The physicians discouraged her. "Almost every single doctor I talked to said something like, 'It's not worth it anymore because it's too expensive.'" Those physicians were on the other side—they had experienced medical training and practice, and many had borrowed heroic sums of money to become experienced—but Sarah was determined to see for herself. She persevered all the way into medical school, only to face her own doubts. Now that she is experiencing the amount of work medical training takes, the circumstances of those discouraging doctors seem more poignant. "How much training goes into that doctor who's like, 'I can't do this shit anymore? I got to get out of here?'"

"The further into debt I get, the more it upsets me. And the more I feel like the expectation is for me to live a life I don't really want to live, the more that it upsets me."

She cannot leave, so she must learn to take on the workload that clinics and hospitals expect.

"I'm too far along, I need this degree at this point. No matter what I do, if I don't end up practicing medicine, I need to have a degree because having half a medical degree is all for shit. You can't do anything with that." Sarah entered medicine because it opened doors and opportunities. "I got into this because there are a lot of things you can do with a medical degree. You can teach, you can do public policy. I thought, 'This is probably safe because there is such a broad range of work that I'm interested in doing, and I can switch if I get bored or whatever.'" The constraint she feels now is not the number of options she might have but the ways in which those options are affected by her financial realities. The possibilities no longer seem endless. The costs do, so the salary matters. "I didn't get into this even considering the salary that I would make. Now it's become a point of contention for me."

. . .

Few physicians admit they enter medicine because it is the most lucrative of the helping professions. But the money and the status are surely part of the reason why medicine remains so attractive; becoming a physician is a lucrative dream that has become the most reliable way to join the 1 percent, even for physicians in the lowest-paid specialties.

Back in the 1970s, the median starting salary of a psychiatrist in academic medicine was $17,000, still in the same neighborhood as the $15,970 median salary of an American public school teacher. By the late 1990s, the median starting salary of a psychiatrist in academic medicine was $69,000, still in the same part of town as the median salary of the contemporary public school teacher, $59,924. By the time Sarah entered medical school, the median starting salary for an academic psychiatrist was $182,000, a different zip code from the teacher's declining median salary of $58,950. And if, by chance, that psychiatrist became the chair of her department, with a median salary of $448,000, they essentially lived in a separate country from schoolteachers [86, 87, 88].

. . .

There are, of course, many variables.

The specialty matters. A specialty like psychiatry is among the lowest paid. Primary care is one the few specialties that falls below psychiatry, and it is falling lower. When Dr. Adams was graduating from residency, the difference in lifetime earnings between a primary care physician and a specialty physician was $3.5 million [89]; it has only grown since.

In the salary reports documenting this split, gender matters too. Within academic medicine, which itself pays less than private practice, the median salary for entry-level physicians is $207,800 for female physicians and $247,900 for male physicians. The differences are only partly explained by the different specialties women and men enter. Physicians in fields like family medicine, general internal medicine, pediatrics, and psychiatry often earn less than the median; these specialties typically attract more women. Physicians in procedural fields like anesthesiology, orthopedic surgery, and interventional radiology often earn more than the median; these specialties typically attract more men [87].

The cost matters. Before applying to medical school, most students complete a four-year undergraduate degree whose cost outpaces inflation. But many students, like Sarah, finish college before completing the requisite premed courses. Students like Sarah can complete the classes one at a time, or in one of the nation's hundreds of postbaccalaureate premedical programs. The postbac premed route, as students call it, is a structured race, usually lasting a year or two, that accelerates medical school entry. Many universities consider the programs as revenue centers because they charge full-tuition prices for entry-level science courses taught by grad students. Add up the cost of those courses, taking the MCAT, and applying for med school, and the average med student owes tens of thousands of dollars on the day med school begins. It wasn't always so expensive.

Med school cost Dr. Boyle $1,000 a year. Even when Dr. Adams started twenty years ago, the median annual cost of attending an in-state public school was $11,511, and that for a private school was $29,748. In twenty years' time, the cost of public medical schools increased 240 percent, and that of private schools increased 112 percent, far exceeding inflation [82]. And those estimates do not include cost of living, including bills for food, shelter, and childcare.

The debt matters. National surveys show that relative debt (i.e., owing more or less than your med school classmates) effects medical students more than absolute debt (i.e., the amount of money you owe). As relative debt increases, students are more likely to report delaying marriage, children, and homeownership [90]. Debt delays lives as much as it alters careers. And it keeps growing, with medical school educational debt increasing an average of 6 percent annually since 1992. Today, the average educational debt of a graduating medical student is $190,000 [91].

The average cloaks inequity. As the average indebtedness of med school graduates is growing, more than a quarter of students graduate without any medical education debt, and those graduates are concentrated in high-income specialties like dermatology and radiology, where salaries can easily be double those of a psychiatrist or primary care physician [92]. This means that the cost of medical school has reinforced inequity, concentrating medical school graduates among people from wealthy backgrounds and the graduates from the wealthiest backgrounds into the highest-income specialties. Hence, as medical school costs have grown during the twenty-first century, the number of medical school entrants from diverse racial backgrounds and lower income quintiles has declined [92]. Today, only one in twenty matriculating medical students comes from the bottom 20 percent of parental incomes. One in five matriculating medical students comes from the highest 20 percent, but a full two in three matriculating medical students come from the highest 40 percent of parental incomes [93]. When experts map the country's applicants, they see that young people from low-income counties are increasingly less likely to apply to medical school than young people from high-income counties [94].

Medical training fancies itself as egalitarian—every student gets the same curriculum, and every resident is paid the same across specialties—but our training system drives inequality. American physicians are the highest paid in the world even as they, like other higheducation elites, have become more politically progressive [95]. Physicians have become literally invested in a system whose most consistent result is the generation of wealth for its leaders. By participating in the system, physicians build the inequality they say they want to address.

Asking questions about how and why physicians generate their wealth might be the most invasive questions a physician could ask. Sarah asks those questions. She asks about how she is trading time for (eventual) money and whether it is worth it. "That upsets me. And then somehow that gets translated to how much money I make." It discomfits Sarah to have a day job enforcing the kind of inequities she wants to eliminate. She worries that physicians are more effective at caring for their own money than for their patients or themselves, but she is in so deep that she must kill her own number first.

Chapter 15

CENTURY WOMEN

$\mathcal{D}$R. ANNA-LISA MUNSON is doing more than her part to realize a new future for medicine. Munson typically sees twelve patients in the morning and twelve more in the afternoon. Many physicians find that supervising even one med student during a busy clinic is too much work. Munson leans in, supervising multiple LIC students in her outpatient pediatric clinic. The clinic opens its doors to patients every weekday at 7:30 a.m. and is typically busy from the moment the doors open. Today, the city's roads are covered with overnight ice, and so many patients have canceled that the clinic itself feels like it is struggling to wake up. The first patient does not even make it to her clinic room until 8:30 a.m.

Aspen, a two-month-old infant, is here for a follow-up visit. Right after birth, the hospitals' pediatricians recorded a hip click, an audible sound from an infant's ligaments. A hip click can be normal right after birth, but if it lingers, it could be a sign that an infant's hip socket doesn't fully cover the ball of the femur. Munson will make the final determination, but Megan Kalata will try first. If normal, Aspen will go on her way; if abnormal, Aspen will be fitted for a harness to train her femur into its socket.

Megan reviews Aspen's measurements, plots them on a growth curve, and enters the examination room. The walls of the square-shaped room are covered with cheery decals of trees and birds, and its examination materials are all child sized. Aspen's full-sized father sits cross-legged on a tiny bench, looking like a giant in a dollhouse. He is dressed in all black—an Obey sweatshirt and stiff Levi's, cuffed to break just so over black Air Force 1s—accompanied by the new car seat and diaper bag of a first-time father. Aspen's mother sits nearby, twisting her task chair side to side. She is also dressed in all black, with green glass gauges in her ears, tattooed birds flying up the side of her neck, and a maroon knitted hairband crowned with a snowflake pattern. She holds Aspen, naked except for a pink blanket and diaper.

The seats are all taken, so Megan stands next to the exam table and asks the parents about sleeping, eating, and diapering. The habits of an infant can set them on the path to a flourishing life. Megan wants to reinforce healthy habits, so she reassures the parents about sleep habits, green poo, and two soft spots instead of one.

Aspen's mother places her daughter on the exam table. Megan begins her exam by raising the pitch of her voice. "Hi, peanut." Megan peers inside Aspen's ears with an otoscope.

"Big bright light." Megan examines Aspen's eyes with an ophthalmoscope.

She encourages the child (and herself), saying, "Good job."

"Strong heart." Megan listens to Aspen's heart with a stethoscope.

"Can I feel your belly?"

"Good grip."

"Check your hips."

"Hi. What's happening? So much is happening."

"Good job, peanut. You're perfect."

The parents draw her attention to a little patch of dry skin on the baby's cheek. Megan peers at the patch before exiting the room to present Aspen to Munson.

. . .

All the students Munson is teaching in clinic are women.

The students believe that the future of medicine is female. They imagine a time when women will achieve equal pay, promotions, and positions. They imagine a version of medical training and practice that is less of a ladder up and more of an evened field. When they look around, Denver Health seems like the place to realize that future: 72 percent of its employees and 60 percent of its physicians are women. The chief executive, medical, and financial officers are women, and so is the chair of its board of directors.

Nationwide, they also see the future arriving. In the 1970s, about 10 percent of American medical students were women. By the 1990s, it was about 40 percent. By the 2020s, women made up 51 percent of medical school applicants, 48 percent of medical school graduates, and 46 percent of residents. They show out, proving again and again that women are more than capable of being physicians. They demonstrate equivalent performance on preliminary work, entrance exams, basic science coursework, clinical work, licensure exams, residencies, and clinical practice. But the students see that women make up only 41 percent of faculty, 25 percent of full professors, and 18 percent of department chairs and deans [96].

Among the physicians at Denver Health, they see that women were less likely to lead a department, practice a procedural discipline, or achieve a full professorship. They see that women are more likely than men to care for children and women [97]. They see that women still experience the constrictions of a professionalized medicine designed for men. They see that some women physicians find it hard to meet an equally educated partner, or even someone who wants an educated partner. Hence, they see that women are still, like the pioneering female physicians before them, creating institutions within institutions through personal connections.

. . .

"She is here for a well-child check." Megan is telling Munson about Aspen.

"The parent's only concern is a dry spot on the cheek, which worsened with the cold weather. She washes her cheek with a warm washcloth. She uses either a scented Johnson & Johnson's lotion or an unscented Burt's Bees lotion. She is formula feeding, four ounces, every four hours. Eight diapers, with one soft bowel movement, a day. Sleeps in a co-sleeping bassinet. They say she is developmentally appropriate, cooing, trying tummy time. As far as physical exam, I could not appreciate the hip click."

Munson nods—no harness for Aspen—while Megan continues.

"She has a small patch of dry skin on her cheek, so I think switching to an unscented lotion would be a good idea."

Munson nods again. Unscented lotion will be preferred. Then she adds, "We could also think about a little bit of hydrocortisone. Also, there was some concern about the mother. Her Edinburgh had been a little high. Unfortunately, we don't have behavioral health here today. Let me review her records. Were they good with shots?"

Megan winces. "Oh, I didn't ask about that."

Munson nods, turns to her MA (medical assistant), and asks if the parents will accept vaccines; the MA says yes.

Munson and Megan return to the exam room. Munson takes the chair next to the computer and starts easy, with recommendations to switch lotions and try hydrocortisone. Now the hard questions: Megan asks about the mother's postpartum blues. "Are you still enjoying seeing the nurse partnership?"

The patient nods. "I am. It's really helped."

"And how do you feel you're doing? I noticed you felt a little overwhelmed on one of the postpartum depression scales, the Edinburgh."

"I get a little overwhelmed sometimes. I'm not worried about her. I just get a little sad sometimes."

Munson offers maternal assurance and medical resources, examines Aspen, offers a little more professional sympathy, schedules the next appointment, and heads to her next room.

There are more patients to see, more work to do in realizing the female future.

Munson personally knows the obstacles her female students will face: the people who will discourage them because of their gender, the people who will make sexual comments, the spouses who will expect them to be responsible for more of the childcare and the housework because it is women's work.

More patients arrive. Munson is measured, wisely reassuring children and parents alike, moving easily among interview, examination, and procedure. Megan stays engaged throughout, projecting calm and confidence, never fumbling interviews or falling into medical jargon.

Solomon is an infant with a granuloma, a little walled-off pocket of inflammation, in his belly button. Megan asks about Solomon's daily habits in a structured way that leads his parents through the developmental highlights: feeding (bottled breast milk every two to three hours), toileting (five to six diapers with mustard-seed-like excrement and eight wet diapers), sleeping (not much). Megan examines Solomon. Solomon urinates; Megan is understanding. Solomon sneezes; Megan offers a bless you. Solomon cries; Megan offers a soothing apology.

She returns to Munson and presents Solomon, and then they return to resolve his granuloma. Megan watches, hands behind her back, as Munson administers silver nitrate to the patient's umbilicus. Munson explains the treatment to the mother and the procedure to Megan as she performs it. "We'll have more of these over the year. I'll do this one. You'll do the next one."

It is a layered promise. They will learn together. They will build the female future, where women are not just patients of medicine but its students and teachers, teaching and learning in ways that embody values different from those of medicine's old hierarchies.

. . .

Hiding in plain sight is that the past was female too; Denver Health was built on the labors of women. In the hospital's basement, three eponymous conference rooms—Nightingale, Osler, and Sabin—host every large educational gathering on the campus. Most attendees probably get the references to Florence (Lady of the Lamp) Nightingale, the British statistician who founded modern nursing, and William (the Saint) Osler, the Canadian physician who reformed medical education. After all, Nightingale and Osler are the most iconic modern nurse and physician, respectively.

Few recognize Sabin. If they do, they probably think that it is a reference to Albert Sabin and his oral polio vaccine. But the room is named for Florence Sabin, the native Coloradoan who was acclaimed as its Woman of the Twentieth Century but is now largely forgotten. Sabin was more responsible than the lamp or the saint, Nightingale or Osler, for the particular shape of Denver Health. Sabin gave the place its form. Sabin gave the place the possibility that its future could be female.

Sabin was born in a mining town 40 miles west of Denver in 1871, five years before the territory earned statehood. When the girls were old enough for school, their frontier family came down the hill to the city. (Such as it was, the Sabins kept cows three blocks north of the state's capital building.) Their frontier home was soon fractured. Nine days after delivering a son, Florence's mother died of sepsis—a nineteenth-century death that would in the next century be preventable. But at the time it left Florence motherless, and her prospector father sent Florence and her sister Mary back east for a Yankee education.

Florence showed a keen appreciation for the Progressive Era's version of the Protestant work ethic: public service, formal education, rationalized vocations. The intersection of these ethics was the ever more scientific, professionalized practice of medicine. And for a woman with aspirations, that meant not a frontier apprenticeship with a practicing physician but the pursuit of a formal degree at Johns Hopkins, where she could learn from Sir William Osler himself, the very model for the *Flexner Report* and, subsequently, for all twentieth-century physicians.

Osler's Hopkins sought men, but they were required to tolerate women. Prominent female benefactors had supported Hopkins during its founding, and through their insistence, Hopkins was more welcoming, begrudgingly, to women than many other medical schools. Sabin was a member of the school's third coed class and lived in the women's dormitory; peers called it the "Hen House." Many women—like Gertrude Stein, a year behind Sabin—left school without degrees. Sabin endured and excelled, finishing third in her class. Class rank determined appointments to the postgraduate residency spots in the hospital's three disciplines—gynecology, medicine, and surgery. Sabin chose the most prestigious, medicine, becoming one of the first women to train under Osler. One year proved enough. Sabin completed an Osler year but passed on further clinical training [98, 99, 100].

Sabin returned to the laboratory and found a mentor in the chair of anatomy, Dr. Franklin P. Mall, who was more welcoming to women. Sabin was a model pupil, publishing an atlas of the medulla—a literal textbook of the body—the very year she completed her internship [101] and a groundbreaking study of the lymphatic system a few years later [102].

Sabin excelled at research. As a professor, she taught that medicine was a technical vocation you undertook with the dedication of a religious calling. Sabin wanted women to follow her to its very pinnacle: research careers. She never married, never mothered, and became a teacher who demanded that her students similarly give their lives to the profession, discouraging female medical students from believing they could have a family life while doctoring [100].

. . .

Megan moves on, seeing a 3-year-old whose sister she also follows on her continuity panel. Megan knows the family well, so she sees the patient alone, charming the child along the way. When she leaves the room, the child shares the smile she withheld at the beginning of the encounter. By 9:20 a.m., Megan has reunited with Munson. Munson sits at one of the workstations clustered in the middle of the clinic. MAs and MDs sit together. The MAs wear blue cotton hospital scrubs and chat with each other in Spanish. Their desks double as supply cabinets for the children's books and blankets they distribute. The MDs dress business casual and speak with each other in English. They cover their desks with textbooks and snapshots and drawings from their children.

Today's pace is slower than usual, so Munson teaches more as they chat. It is not one of the hierarchical lessons favored in the old model—where a senior physician, usually a man, publicly asked questions to stump trainees at every level of the hierarchy, to gauge medical knowledge and reinforce a student's place at the bottom of the ladder, a practice called "pimping"—but a personal conversation about the best way to help the child Megan just saw. The just-in-time teaching session ends when an MA rooms the next patient, Jesus, a 4-year-old Latino boy in an astronaut-themed gown.

Jesus is crying on the exam table, while his elders stand around him. Megan approaches him with a picture book. Jesus flips through it but is reluctant to give up his tears. As he fidgets on the examination table, his mother says, "We can't fool him, he started crying as soon as we turned into the parking lot." His father stands across the room. Megan sits at the computer station, but instead of turning it on, she addresses the mother.

The mother denies any concerns about his health, so Megan asks after their habits. Jesus likes being read to. He struggles with scissors. He likes grilled cheese. Jesus pipes in, saying "grilled cheese" repeatedly for the next several minutes, but Megan presses her questions. Jesus dislikes broccoli, tolerates cauliflower, and likes carrots. He eats hamburgers and hot dogs but never the buns. He drinks two to three sippy cups of milk nightly, Capri Sun twice a day, Crystal Light throughout the day, and occasionally diet soda.

Megan listens, encourages the mother to discontinue sugary drinks, and logs on to the computer. Megan reviews Jesus's growth chart with his parents, reinforcing why he needs to avoid sugary drinks. Sensing the mother's engagement, Megan expands the conversation into a discussion of dental care. Jesus dislikes dentists almost as much as doctors. At the word "dentist," crying overtakes him, and Jesus slips off the exam table like he is trying to escape. But his wandering around the small room only brings him closer to Megan. Megan resumes her review with his mother: toileting, sleeping, reading.

Megan washes her hands. She asks Jesus's mother why she is declining a flu shot. "I think he's healthy and I give him a multivitamin." Megan tries, "I think it's great that he's healthy, but he'll be around people who aren't healthy, and it is one of the best ways to protect him." The mother declines, saying she will accept only the other vaccines, so Megan moves on to the exam. Jesus's crying accelerates. Megan engages him, talking about how strong he is, asking him where his heart is, allowing him to hold her stethoscope, and asking what she will hear in his tummy. She soothes Jesus long enough to examine his body and then exits to present his case to Munson.

. . .

Women have faced many discouragements in the house of medicine. Leading physicians once claimed that the only way a woman could practice medicine is if they gave up being a woman. Menstruation, they asserted, rendered women simply too irregular. You could be an irregular woman or a regular physician; pick one. The metaphorical doors to medical practice were barred until 1835, when the sisters Harriot and Sarah Hunt became the first American women to successfully practice medicine. Dr. Sarah Hunt practiced only a few years, leaving medicine to marry and raise six children. She picked motherhood; her sister picked medicine. Dr. Harriot Hunt stayed in the field and secured a series of firsts. In 1852, she (along with Nancy Talbot Clark) became the first American woman to seek certification from a state medical society. In 1860, Dr. Hunt celebrated a silver anniversary, marking her twenty-five years of union with medical practice, of being wedded to work. Despite her devotion, doors remained barred; Hunt was denied admission to Harvard despite a letter of recommendation from Oliver Wendell Holmes himself.

Women like Harriot Hunt found that they were better off relying only on other women for encouragement, and female supporters raised money and built institutions where they could train and practice. Nineteenth-century women's medical colleges—in Boston, but also in Atlanta, Baltimore, Chicago, Cincinnati, Cleveland, Kansas City, New York City, Philadelphia, and St. Louis—were separate, but unequal, facilities whose very existence testified to the ability and determination of women [19]. Through such efforts, the number of women physicians rose from about two thousand to about seven thousand between 1880 and 1900 [15, p. 92].

In her history of female physicians, Regina Morantz-Sanchez observed that individual women built spaces for each other within the institutions of American medicine. Some of those spaces came at the expense of other women, like the midwives whose artisanal practices were displaced by physicians. Some of these spaces were made by the state, as land-grant and public universities were quicker to admit female medical students than the private universities favored by philanthropists. Some of those spaces were at the expense of domestic life, as women were counseled that they could not be a wife and mother as well as a doctor. Some of those spaces were stereotyped, as women were typecast as nurturers. Some of those spaces were proscribed for women, as they were allowed to enter obstetrics, pediatrics, primary care, and public health but not procedural specialties. Some of those spaces belonged to them, as they created institutions of their own. "The overall effect" of professionalism, which required formal, extended, university-based training to enter medicine, was, in the words of Morantz-Sanchez, "to constrict women's activity as physicians, and to confine their participation to particular specialties already implicitly agreed upon in the nineteenth century" [15, p. 234].

Constricted and confined by outmoded models, American female physicians often found themselves being asked if they were physicians or women. Osler was a progressive, but a patriarchal one, declaring that there were three kinds of people: men, women, and women physicians [15, p. 142]. Osler's quip was one of many reminders to women physicians of the dilemmas they faced. Sabin tried to outrun the dilemma by taking Osler's advice to its logical conclusion. Osler delayed marriage; Sabin never married. Osler became a physician-educator; Sabin became a physician-scientist. Osler counseled day-tight compartments; Sabin made hers into a leading laboratory.

Sabin lived out Osler's counsel, but male physicians haltered her ascension anyway. When her mentor, Dr. Mall, died, Sabin was passed over for the chairmanship of the anatomy department. One of her former students received the chair she had sought. Dr. Lewis Weed was soon named dean of the entire medical school, directing it for decades. Weed grew up in elite private institutions—Yale, Hopkins, Harvard— and ascended to their leadership. Sabin settled for a lesser chair, of the histology department. And while she became the first female full professor at Hopkins, she was never allowed to vote as a member of the faculty, and she left Hopkins when Weed became dean.

She joined the Rockefeller Institute in New York City, where the polymath became the delight of New York's academic society, albeit one who still had her clothes made by a Denver dressmaker [99, p. 129]. Those dresses helped maintain her connection to her home, and when Sabin eventually retired, she left New York City and lived with her beloved sister Mary in an apartment a mile from Denver Health.

It was a quiet retirement, until her home state realized her abilities. In December 1944, Colorado's governor was preparing for the eventual return of World War II veterans to civilian life. At the encouragement of a local reporter, the governor put Sabin in charge of improving her native state's health, an opportunity to realize her vision of medical study, which began by creating detailed textbooks of the body's brain stem and lymphatic system, expanded to the treatment of individual disease, and was later fulfilled in the prevention of social diseases.

Osler is better remembered, but Sabin is a better future. Osler taught the textbook of the body, while Sabin taught the two textbooks, body and community.

On March 29, 1946, she organized a meeting of civic leaders and challenged them. "What are we all going to do together about Colorado's health conditions? We must develop a program to give to people so that their interest, now aroused, will not die" [99, pp. 155–56]. Sabin knew what she wanted to do together, drafting eight legislative bills for public health, colloquially called the "Sabin Health Bills," five for building health infrastructure and three for addressing specific diseases. The bills established the state's public health department, as well as county and city health departments; provided funds for the building of hospitals; appropriated funds for the medical school; and increased the hospital payment for indigent care by 50 percent [103]. Sabin toured the state's sixty-three counties, speaking to any group she could, and won passage of seven of the eight bills.

Then Sabin improved the state's capital city, taking over the management of what was then called the City of Denver's Health and Charities department. The institution that would become Denver Health was, at the time, a city agency under Health and Charities' aegis. The hospital was called Denver General—people joked that its initials DG stood for *Don't Go*, the kind of slur often placed on facilities for the marginalized. Sabin turned it into a teaching hospital like Hopkins, but with a public health focus that made community-wide impacts on health.

Sabin turned Denver Health into the place where medical research passed from the study of disease to the study of health through the work of education, where a student could learn from the textbook of the body and textbook of the community. Sabin made it an institution that would be led by generations of women, even as it remained a place where women were still trying to realize a truly female future, a place where they could be physicians and partners and parents, if they desired. It was the kind of future Munson was fighting for, on a snowy morning, with Megan.

. . .

"Jesus has no concerns," Megan tells Munson. "I showed them the growth curve and where his weight is above his height. It sounds like he actually likes vegetables, but he mostly eats grilled cheese, cheeseburgers, and a lot of sugary drinks." Megan reviews Jesus's dental health, sleep (his parents cannot afford a separate bed for him), school (mostly at home, seeking entry into a free childcare program). Megan summarizes the physical exam: "everything is normal, except for his weight." Megan discusses the mother's reluctance to accept a flu shot. Munson takes a stand. Munson believes in vaccines.

"I have started telling mothers about patients who have died from the flu this year."

At 10:27 a.m., Munson and Megan enter Jesus's exam room. He is still crying. He points to his foot and insists she listen to his feet with her stethoscope. Munson offers to do so. While he is climbing onto the exam table, Munson washes her hands and tries her flu shot gambit. The mother declines again. Munson demurs and begins her examination. At Jesus's insistence, she listens to his right toe with a stethoscope. She has Jesus count backward from ten. In between descending numbers, he keeps asking, in a panicked voice, "Are we done?" Thanks to Munson's experienced exam, they quickly are.

Outside the room, Munson visits her MA. "Jesus is ready for his vaccines and out of his skull." The MA keeps her calm, gathers her supplies, and quickly administers the vaccines to the crying Jesus. Minutes later, Jesus departs with his mother.

. . .

In some ways, Sabin is a clear model for Dr. Munson, Megan, and other female physicians. In other ways, they are still fighting against her idea that medicine must be the sole focus of a good physician. Though most would accept that women can be a physician and physicians can be women, medicine remains so hierarchical that, even today, few women rise to the heights Sabin achieved without making some of the sacrifices she counseled.

A century after Sabin, most of the LIC students are women. The program's leader and many of the core faculty are women as well. Their abilities have been demonstrated in course after course, examination after examination, encounter after encounter. And yet, most can tell stories of conflict between a woman's perceived role and a doctor's perceived role.

Munson sees a few patients on her own. Fluent in French and Spanish, she has many patients from West Africa and Central America.

Mallory Myers arrives at the clinic. One of Mallory's cohort patients is scheduled for a clinic visit, so Mallory arrives early to greet the patient, whom she has seen in acute and chronic settings.

Mallory remembers one of her discouragements as a woman. "A pastor told me that women should not be doctors because they should be wives and mothers, and you can't do both." Ironically, the pastor and Sabin seemed to agree on one point about the physician's vocation: you could not simultaneously be a physician and a parent. Mallory's own mother reassured her with stories of female physicians who both practiced medicine and raised families. The Denver Health faculty assured Mallory that both roles were possible. Most of her supervising physicians were women, and most were also parents, giving Mallory hope that she could be a physician, despite discouragements.

As Munson conducts bilingual visits, Megan sits and considers adding Aspen to her cohort. When Megan meets a patient who might be a good cohort patient, she adds them to her list in the EHR, which alerts her when they are scheduled for a clinic visit, are hospitalized, or otherwise encounter the health system. Megan finds that cohort building also requires building alliances with patients who want to engage with students, so she has gotten better at adopting Munson's encouraging tone when examining children and Munson's consoling words when assuring mothers. Students need those skills to keep patients engaged in treatment because patients often fall out of care.

It happens for Mallory. Her cohort patient has not shown, so Mallory has trekked over in the snow for naught. She looks discouraged, but her face brightens at the sight of an alert from Kris Oatis telling her that another one of her cohort patients, a pregnant woman, is laboring. Mallory trudges through the snow to the hospital so she can examine her. The patient is a first-time mom, so things could move slowly, but Mallory is hopeful to get a delivery.

Munson and Megan work on realizing the female future for medicine, despite the snow and all the other discouragements in their way.

Chapter 16

GRAVE DISEASE

"I WAS FEELING REALLY WEIRD, shaky, hungry, all those symptoms that a medical student gets when they're in the OR." Itzam Marin felt run-down by his surgery immersion, as expected. Since adolescence, Itzam had been a professional—first in football, soon in medicine. Anticipating demanding labor, Itzam attributed his shaking to long hours spent retracting, suctioning, and breathing recirculated air while wearing personal protective equipment. The clinical year can wear you down, just like it can burn you out. Some students shake and somatize, their thoughts jinking from disease to disease, seeking a dramatic explanation for what could be shivering their limbs. Not Itzam. He leaned into his training. He diagnosed himself as not exercising enough for the OR's physical demands.

Attending surgeons saw his shaking and made their own diagnosis: nerves. Some students get anxious in the sterilized space of the operating room. Some students fall out at the sight of the specialized scissors arrayed around an unspeaking patient. Some students shake at the thought of a patient's airway being controlled by a machine. Some students sweat through their surgical rotation, eager for the day when they can leave the operating room. Not Itzam. He wanted to make his mark in the OR as a surgeon. He was sure it wasn't nervous shaking.

. . .

Medical students are famous for diagnosing themselves. In libraries and lecture halls, they learn about conditions that can sicken suddenly or stun by degrees. They memorize the signs of obscure diseases. They learn about how a seemingly random constellation of symptoms can herald a life-altering illness. They look at themselves. *A bump on my neck, my recent weight loss, a night of sweating.* With symptoms like that, a first-year medical student can conclude that they have the miliary tuberculosis their professor has been lecturing them about.

It's a well-known stage on the road to becoming a physician: a few months as a hypochondriacal medical student [104]. Some med students go so far as to invent their own conditions—one physician-author of a novel about medical school wrote of Dreadful Hoof Dismay, Atrocious Pancreas Oh, Crispy Lung Surprise, and Chronic Kidney Doom [105]. Hypochondriasis is a med student's way of unconsciously defending against all the varieties of illness they are learning about, as well as the fourth *D* lurking behind Dr. Adams's warning.

Most medical students abandon hypochondriasis right around the time they receive their visible defenses, the stiff white coats that empower medicals students to enter clinical spaces on the doctor's side of the physician-patient divide. But it is effortful to keep coats white while contacting the blood, bile, and bodily fluids of patients.

The literal effort occurs in the hospital's basement laundry room, where all traces of bodily fluids are removed. The laundry's workers clean the bedsheets and surgical drapes that patients stain and bloody. They clean the white coats of physicians too. But the patient's garments are folded by machines. The laundry's workers press white coats by hand on a prewar machine whose model name is hand-painted on the side in shadowed letters: PROSPERITY. The machine's heat and heft keep physician's coats shiningly white, restoring their veneer of perfectionistic prosperity. Everything about medical training—the years of schooling, the selection of the able, the intolerance of failure—maintains that veneer and marks a physician out from a particular group of others: from the people who are sick.

Physicians wear white coats; patients wear hospital gowns. Physicians treat illness; patients suffer illness. These divisions defend doctors against the realization that they, and everyone they love, will eventually suffer illness or injury, be diminished into being a patient.

The marking out of a future doctor from their patient occurs during the clinical year.

At the beginning of the year, the students identify with the patients. *That bed looks lumpy, the food smells rotten, and the doctors intrude rudely.* On rounds, they think with the patients, aware of their concerns.

It usually does not last.

By the end of a rotation, they identify with the physicians. *They never take their meds, they never follow the dressing orders, and the patients delay healing.* On rounds, they start to think with the physicians, aware of their concerns.

That lasts—unless a diagnosis intrudes into a medical student's own training.

. . .

Health systems prefer dramatic diagnoses. Hospitals make money on crashing cars, ruptured organs, sprawling tumors, and severed limbs. They lose money on skin ailments, joint pains, and back pains, even though those are the most common reasons people visit physicians. In the quiet of exam rooms, far away from the services advertised on billboards, patients bring these ordinary trials before their physicians, laying their concerns out like a fleece before a minor god whose miracles are poultices, potions, and pills rather than fire from a rock. When you read med school applications, aspirants to the house of medicine write about stemming pandemics, developing breakthroughs, and ending inequities. If the genre allowed candor, applicants would talk about back pain in their admission essays.

To prepare the LIC students to receive humble offerings, Dr. Jennifer Stichman is leading a Thursday afternoon classroom session about the venerable and vulnerable lumbar area of the spine. Stichman strides in on camel-colored suede clog heels, held over her bare feet with a single strap. She wears a beige and black dress with geometric patterns that repeat and intersect and follow her body's line of action as she moves about the room, distributing her no-drama handout: "Evaluation of Low Back Pain in Adults." As she prepares, the students are sharing pictures on phones, snacking from shared bags, and laughing about bodily fluids. Pus, phlegm, pericardial effusions. So many fluids, presenting when least welcome, but helpfully revealing what ails a patient.

Stichman steps to the whiteboard and quickly writes out a clinical bullet point. *66 yo man. Stoic. Reluctant talker. Lives in a camper. Food insecurity. 20 lb. weight loss.* Lifting her hand from the board, she turns to the students and asks what they want to know. They snap to attention and offer questions. On the whiteboard, Stichman organizes the resulting answers in the pattern that is becoming second nature to the students: *CC, HPI, ROS, SH, FH, PE*—abbreviations for components of the H&P, history and physical, that gradually translates a patient's complaints into a physician's story. Some students race to the story's conclusion, expecting the punchline to be cancer, because why else would an American man lose 20 pounds unintentionally?

Stichman shakes off the shortcut and the easy answer. Moving her dry-erase marker confidently across the whiteboard, she fills it with medical abbreviations while speaking aloud the many Latinate words of a rheumatologist. She enunciates—*tendonitis, enthesitis, circinate balanitis, pyoderma gangrenosum*—with purpose. When students share her language, trading the colloquial "sausage toes" for the medical "dactylitis," her whole freckled face expresses approval and the great mass of red hair pulled loosely into a halo curl above it shakes in confident appreciation. She wants the students to document in medical language but to speak with patients in a language they understand. She wants code-switchers, doctors who can talk both to each other and to patients.

A student proposes to ask a patient, "Do you have any perineal pain?"

"That's a medical term that patients do not know."

"Groin pain?"

"That's better, but even that is a word that not all patients know. What do all patients know? A friend of mine taught me to ask: 'When you wipe, can you feel it?'"

The students laugh but press on.

"MSK pain?"

"You don't get to say MSK to a rheumatologist."

"Muscular strain?"

"Muscular strain?" Stichman shifts her head from side to side before settling in the midline. "I can accept that." She writes "muscular strain" on the board, because it has sufficient specificity for physician-physician communication.

The students focus on pathophysiology, asking classic ROS—review of systems—questions that screen for dysfunction in the major organ systems. At one point, Stichman chides them for not asking about SH and FH—social and family history—saying, "I know you care about that."

Together, the students and Stichman generate a differential diagnosis for the patient's back pain, a list of possible causes: cauda equina syndrome, spinal cord injury, cancer metastases of many flavors (breast, prostate, kidney, colon, lung, thyroid), herniated or degenerated disc, spinal stenosis, infection, osteomyelitis, muscular strain, renal stones, abdominal aortic aneurysm, and pancreatitis, atrocious and otherwise.

And so it goes, with Stichman leading the students in a merry discussion of the ways the body bends, breaks, and leaks, as well as how a physician can suss out the cause through the PE—the physical examination. Maggie Kriz proposes checking for an anal wink.

Stichman replies, "What is the anal wink? Is that the same as the digital rectal exam? The wink is when you touch the skin, and the anus puckers. I think you might elicit an anal wink if you performed a digital rectal exam, but you need to be careful. They are different." Stichman admits no fear of the body. For example, after Adams's appendix was surgically removed, Stichman gifted Adams a plush stuffed appendix instead of flowers. She is the kind of person for whom being careful is about performing the correct physical exam maneuver, no matter how invasive. She is the kind of person we call a physician.

To help her students become the same kind of person, she asks which diagnostic studies the students would order. They summon up an acronymic blizzard of labs to perform on the patient (CBC, BMP, TSH, U/A, ESR, Alk phos) and imaging procedures (CXR, MRI T-Spine versus CT Spine), but Stichman stops the diagnostic storm. She will allow a test only if a student can explain what they are really seeking from each test.

. . .

What Itzam wanted was a diagnosis of his own. Even after he left surgery, the shaking persisted. During his internal medicine immersion, he finally admitted that it was a problem beyond insufficient exercise.

"I was feeling bad through the whole of medicine. I remember holding my hands, to see my notes during rounds, and the notes would be floppy and illegible. It was hard for me to write, too, because you need to write really small on your papers. You cannot fit all the HPI on your presentation notes, especially when it's your first time. I was like, 'Something is definitely off.'"

But what? Itzam did not know. He put his white coat back on and went back to the wards.

. . .

The grown-up version of med school admission essays are physician memoirs, and such memoirs often hinge on the author's discovery that a white coat is not an immunity cloak. Patients puke up on, piss on, and pass out over physicians, but somehow many physicians have an unspoken belief that disease will pass them by. The white coat stays clean, so its wearer stays well. *PROSPERITY.*

Medical training maintains the defense. The long hours—which stretch quickly into years of physical demands and emotional commitments—assume health. When we imagine a physician, most people cannot picture a blind, deaf, or disabled medical student. Medical training imperiously presumes an able body.

The cultural expectation in medicine is that a physician will not be sick and that if a doctor gets sick, they will stoically work though. A doctor takes no sick days. Researchers who study what they call "workplace presenteeism" across professions find that physicians are the most likely to show up at work with an infectious disease [106]. When researchers survey physicians and other clinicians, they find that while nineteen of twenty clinicians know that working while sick risks the health of their patients, five of six clinicians have worked sick at least once in the past year, and almost one of ten reported working sick at least five times in the past year. They came to work despite diarrhea, fever, and respiratory symptoms. And physicians were more likely than other clinicians to come to work sick. When asked why, they said that they did not want to let the profession down. They are physicians, not patients. Their colleagues and patients needed them. There was no staff to take their place if they called in sick. They feared being ostracized if they did so [107].

When backup is available for sick days, physicians call it Jepo, short for jeopardy. Some other physician is on backup call, available to be pulled from their own work to cover yours. If you call in sick, the backup physician is jeopardized. You can call jeopardy on occasion without consequence. If you call jeopardy on every occasion, you develop a reputation. Best not to call and jeopardize your career. Better to work and jeopardize your patients, to be what researchers call a "hazardous hero" [108].

Physicians too often even raise their children on the Jepo model. They are reluctant to keep sick children home from school. They have been known to dose their kids with just the right amount of ibuprofen to keep fevers at bay long enough for them to make it to the hospital, so that they can finish rounds before the pharmacological half-life crests. Doing so may make them bad parents, but it has the reputation of making them good physician parents. All of this is to say that stoic medical culture—and the systems that depend on it—encourages showing up sick.

Physicians swap war stories about working while ill. Dr. Adams gets a stuffed appendix because she was politicking for funding soon after her own appendix was removed. She and Stichman have an emergency medicine colleague who is famous for having performed a cricothyrotomy, a lifesaving incision in the neck of a patient who could not breathe, between the forceful breaths of her own labor contractions. Itzam sweated and shook but stayed in the operating rooms and on the wards, looking like an anxious and hungry future physician.

. . .

The psychiatrist Robert Klitzman studied dozens of doctors who experienced a grave disease, such as breast cancer, myocardial infarctions, and HIV. For each, the realization that they could become ill was a surprise. Medicine, Klitzman observed, attracts controlling and conscientious people who are inclined to seek certainty, to seek mastery. Medical training implicitly taught his respondents that illness is something physicians treat and patients suffer. As physicians gain personal experience of illness, they lose their naivete.

Even so, Klitzman's physicians clung to what separated them from "real" patients. They maintained many clinical privileges. They enjoyed easier access to treatment and more treatment options. They understood, at least partially, the treatments available to them. They often treated themselves, from self-diagnosing, like Itzam, to even self-treatment and self-prescribing. When they allowed someone else to treat them, they often selected a physician who was a friend and allowed them more access than most patients.

For all those differences, the experience of sickness softened the dividing line, teaching the physicians the truth of the old saw that a minor illness is only minor if someone else has it. Klitzman's ill physicians simultaneously suffered and learned from being ill. "They learned how patient time, doctor time, and hospital time conflicted; how 'a person waiting is a person suffering'; and how poor access to a doctor can reinforce disturbing feelings of dependency and loss" [109, pp. 125-26].

. . .

On the internal medicine wards, Itzam examined his patient. Insomnia, weight loss, tremor, hyperactivity, sweating. The symptoms all added up to a diagnosis. Itzam recognized the patient's symptoms as signs of Graves's disease, an autoimmune disorder in which immunoglobins are produced that act against a person's thyroid, stimulating hormone receptors and leading to the overproduction of thyroid hormone, which can make the person anxious and hungry. Then, Itzam thought of his own symptoms and realized that he, too, had Graves's disease. Making the diagnosis twice made him, simultaneously, the kind of person who is both a physician and a patient.

But when he told people at the hospital that he had Graves's disease, no one believed him. He was just another medical student diagnosing himself with a disease he had recently studied. He was told it was just his body getting used to the physician's life, growing pains more than a growing disease. When doctors would not listen, Itzam told his wife, Andrea.

"My wife got annoyed at me because I kept bringing up the symptoms, and she told me, 'You need to go to a doctor or, if not, you are not going to talk to me about this anymore.'"

Only his friend, a fellow med student, supported his hunch. After sitting together through a lunchtime thyroid lecture, they were certain. Itzam needed care of his own. Itzam would, for the first time, be a patient. Late on the next afternoon, he checked into the on-campus clinic at the med school. When the nurse practitioner asked the reason for his visit, he proffered an earthy chief complaint that would have made Stichman proud: "I just feel like crap."

His concern was resisted.

"The nurse practitioner was like, 'It seems like you're really stressed and those long hours without sleep in third year can be hard for your body. I want to reassure you that things are okay.'"

Itzam felt like the nurse practitioner wanted to prescribe him some meds to take the edge off. Itzam wanted a thyroid function test, not a Xanax. He could palpate his own thyroid, and what he found there was what worried him. He insisted on the test. After a quick venipuncture, a sample of his serum was off to the lab. While the sample was processing, Itzam went back to the wards, since it would be another day before his results returned. When they arrived, they felt like a kind of victory.

"It was World Cup time. And I got home at 7 a.m. after a 24-hour shift, my wife had the TV on, and Argentina was playing. She is a soccer fan, born and raised in Argentina. By 8 a.m., I received the labs through

MyChart directly into my phone. And with a sense of worry and reassurance, I saw a T4 that was through the roof and a TSH that was super low. I quickly ran through the differential diagnosis in my head, 'Maybe Graves's disease? It can also be DeQervain, hopefully not a hot nodule, those are rare right?'"

He called his friend to tell him about the labs. They crowed that they had suspected the diagnosis and that their suspicions were borne out. His friend shouted over the phone, "I'm never wrong, bro!" and then pivoted to concern: "Are you doing okay, though?"

. . .

Once Itzam became a patient, he acted quickly to secure definitive treatment that would rid his body of Graves's disease. Graves's is one of the hundreds of eponyms in clinical medicine, each bearing testament to the textbook-of-the-body approach to medicine. You discover it, and medicine memorializes you. Some sound charming: *Bell palsy*. Some sound pejorative: *Cryer syndrome*. Some sound like law firms: *Bland-White-Garland syndrome*. Some sound perverse: *Cock peculiar disease*.

The name of Itzam's condition memorializes Dr. Robert James Graves, who described hyperthyroidism in 1853, the last year of his epic nineteenth-century life. He saved a sinking ship. He was falsely imprisoned as a spy. He conducted hospital rounds by candlelight. He stopped a typhus outbreak on the west coast of Ireland. He invented the second hand on watches. But he is remembered for observing the hypothyroidism that, for reasons still unknown, produces the kind of lab results that delighted and concerned Itzam's friend [110].

Itzam earned a direct ticket, thanks to those lab results, to the endocrine clinic for definitive treatment, the intentional dissolution of an internal organ. Itzam saw the very endocrinologist who taught him about the thyroid during the first two years of medical school. Itzam's teacher taught him that the thyroid gland absorbs almost all iodine in the body, and now, as Itzam's physician, he could use this fact. The endocrinologist assured Itzam that he could administer a radioiodine pill that would be so well absorbed by the thyroid gland that it would be ablated, leaving behind an absent space in Itzam's neck.

. . .

Back in the classroom, Itzam answers Stichman's prompts. He explains the lab results—all normal except for a mild vitamin D insufficiency, which provides no diagnostic clarity—and then volunteers his own experience. While the hypothetical diagnostic tests the students suggested where unrevealing and, therefore, probably unnecessary, Itzam explains how the right diagnostic test can distinguish garden-variety medical student nerves from a treatable disease. He tells Stichman and his peers that his own anxiety pointed to something more than an adjustment to the clinical year, which was confirmed after his own labs came back. The labs were decidedly necessary; they revealed Graves's disease. There was a quick cascade from lab result, to diagnosis, to treatment. Treatment was radiofrequency ablation. He offers this information casually, and his classmates receive it the same way. One teases him, asking whether he misses being hyperthyroid.

Itzam rubs the blank space on his neck and admits that he does, at least a little, and the discussion moves on. Stichman guides the students through tests and treatments, until she reaches the reveal of every internist's story: the diagnosis.

Some of the students are distracted by the red herrings in the clinical story. They hear weight loss and back pain and think cancer. Itzam does not. Of all the students in the room, he is the one who reaches the correct diagnosis of Stichman's patient—a fracture from a generalized tonic-clonic seizure—just as he correctly diagnosed himself.

. . .

Itzam learned that being a physician is not easy, but it is always harder to be the patient. The categories collapse in time. All physicians eventually become patients.

Think of Robert Graves. He buried two wives and two children, experienced a profound bout of depression, and developed abdominal cancer. He knew, in his own life, that being a physician afforded thin protection against patienthood. Most physicians experienced morbidity and mortality on a personal level during the era.

So when, during the last decade of Graves's life, the Massachusetts legislature studied the mean age at death of people in various occupations, they found that bank officers outlived everyone, dying between ages 68 and 76. (Damn those bank officers!) Clerks and teachers had the shortest life spans, dying between the ages of 30 and 35. In between the bankers and teachers were the "Blacksmiths, butchers, calico printers, lawyers, hatters, merchants, physicians, and ropemakers," dying between the ages of 50 and 55 [111]. In that era, a physician knew illness and infirmity not just as a professional but as a patient. Just like the blacksmiths and butchers, a physician made himself more vulnerable to various illnesses and injuries when he entered the profession.

By the time Dr. Adams entered medical school in 2000, however, the average age of death for physicians was 70.3 years, which is part of why concerns about physician well-being have lately shifted from infectious diseases to mental illnesses. Physicians were no longer likely to die of the infectious diseases they treated at work. The biggest danger of their work seemed to be burnout, exhaustion from the experience of caring itself [112, 113]. Physicians still died six years shy of the average American, but most physicians experienced a longevity and a health that profoundly delayed their entry into the ranks of patients [112].

Illness arrives for everyone eventually. Early or late, when physicians experience the involuntary discharges of their own body fluids, they must reckon with the limits of their white coat. White coats confer only the illusion of immunity. Illness strips illusions by changing physicians back into patients.

. . .

Illness changed Itzam.

"It really opened my mind," Itzam said. "I used to tell patients, 'Yeah, we're going to get this lab and then we can start the medication if this happens.' When I was a patient, when that was happening to me, all I could think of, even when I was rotating on internal medicine, when I was seeing patients, was 'What does that result say? What's the next step?' I needed to know, to make time to get my pills, make time to get the radioablation. 'How am I going to isolate myself?' That's all I could think of, all I could do."

For a short time after his teacher ablated Itzam's thyroid, Itzam restricted household contact so as not to irradiate his wife. His treatment had the potential to render her infertile.

"I feel pretty lucky that I had the knowledge to understand radioablation. It's so hard for most people to understand. And even I had to look up things about radioablation. Like, 'How soon can I start trying to have kids and all this stuff?'

"It was hard to concentrate because I wasn't myself. Even though Graves's is such an easily treatable disease, that's all I could think of."

He knows his own experience was a good one. Of all the grave diseases that can affect a physician, his is readily treatable. He learned from the experience, becoming more attentive to patients, as well as more resolved to seek his Match in surgery. Still, for the rest of his life he will take a thyroid replacement hormone, a substitute for what the destroyed gland in his neck once made. The mark on his neck would remind him, for the rest of his days, that he was a physician and patient.

Now Itzam wonders if he can learn one more thing from his illness.

Before the clinical year started, he spoke often of how much he admired his wife, Andrea. His classmates said, privately, that he called her his "savior" as often as his "wife." Itzam admired Andrea for her strong personality, strong voice, and strong drive. All her strengths attracted Itzam to Andrea.

During his clinical year, she worked in human resources for a hotel. He saw that physicians were not the only ones who worked long hours. They came home at the same time and returned to work at the same time, but Andrea was the one bringing salary into their household, while he was adding student loans. He felt that Andrea understood that they were delaying gratification, working hard now so that they could build for their future, their own cake and ale years. When important exams appeared on the calendar, Andrea would understand that he had to study, but she would tease him: *You better get a good score.* They wanted good scores, good careers, and, eventually, good children, but the timing changed after Itzam's illness.

"I was the one that had to be convinced a little bit earlier, but it was not hard. We were thinking about this since before med school and we were trying to hit for a year past residency."

Itzam makes it sound as if the real lesson is to partner and parent even while doctoring. He is becoming confident he will be a good physician. He, after all, diagnosed his own disease. It often takes decades for a physician to realize how illness feels differently when experienced by a patient and a physician. Itzam learned another old lesson even before he became a doctor: *Medice, cura te ipsum.* Indeed. Now, Itzam is wondering if it is time to parent as well.

Chapter 17
INSIGNIFICANT OTHERS

$\mathcal{M}$ALLORY MYERS SENSED that a med student's anxiety sometimes signaled affection instead of illness. "I started to suspect something the day before. He and his friend were texting and keeping a secret. I was nervous for him because he was so nervous."

Mallory has a nervous boyfriend. He is a student in the traditional version of med school, thinking of surgery. She is thinking of internal medicine. Both are thinking of each other and wondering if they should tie their fates together in marriage. Every marriage is a union. Medical marriages can be a union of a couple and their careers. A medical couple can tie their fates together as soon as the Match, ensuring that they wind up at the same hospital, in the same city, or at least in the same region. They can even risk going unmatched rather than being separated. Couples Matching adds an extra degree of difficulty to the typically demanding Match. And yet many medical students make the wager. Marrying after the clinical year is a popular timeline for today's medical students. The clinical year is the proving ground, but the last half of the fourth and final year of med school is usually a victory lap and, often, a wedding dance. Somewhere between Match Day and the start of residency, many med students find time to say their I Dos.

. . .

Some students marry before they enter medicine. Sarah Bardwell, Mackenzie Garcia, and Itzam Marin were already married by the beginning of the clinical year. Their questions were more about whether those relationships could endure and when to arrange parenting around their training. Sarah has answers.

At the start of a Thursday class, Sarah shares her news with her classmates: her long-delayed divorce had been finalized. Her classmates celebrate. She now qualifies for Medicaid, like most of her patients. She will no longer receive her ex's mail. She can focus on becoming a physician. Sarah will enter the Match alone.

"My sister has some kids. My mom, and my sister, and the kids, all live at my mom's house, and so I can go over there and hold babies and have little kids sit on my lap." After days and nights with the ill, holding children makes Sarah feel well—"It's the best, very rejuvenating, humanizing experience"—but she rarely thinks of having children of her own.

"I feel like I've passed the point of considering kids. There was a period of my mid-twenties, late twenties when I was really into it. And then I had a failed marriage attempt and went through that grieving process. Now I'm on the other side. I have a bunch of godkids and I'm an auntie, and that role works out really well for me. My work is where I'm invested right now."

. . .

Halfway through the year, the students are into the rhythm of investing in the right now. They have identified their continuity patients, learned to dress in the dark, figured out the location of every bailout bathroom, and restructured their lives around the lives of their patients and preceptors. They now live by the medical clock—arriving early to prepare patients for surgery, staying late to see patients whose problem lists cannot be seized in the clinic, and staying up with patients laboring through the night. They have been sneezed, spat, vomited, peed, and bled on. Each student is figuring out their fluids and their patients, as they figure out how they want to put themselves forward as physicians in the world.

Now Dr. Adams teaches a lesson about how seeing physicians can be bad for the health of patients. Physicians, Adams says, can unintentionally harm a patient. Physicians, Adams teaches, can order too many tests, prescribe too many meds, perform too many procedures, and involve too many other clinicians in ways that harm patients.

Even as they are learning all of what can be done medically, Adams is encouraging the students to narrow their focus to what absolutely needs to be done. "Look for clinical vignettes, for patient stories, about overuse and send me a one-liner of your case. Often, students identify a true error. If you send me a one-liner, I can tell you if you're on the right track. We're looking for times when people do the right thing and it causes harm."

. . .

Adams enjoins the students to follow the ancient injunction *primum non nocere* (first, do no harm). Many medical students are simultaneously answering the family question, *omnia vincit amor* (love conquers all). Virgil was Hippocrates's superior in poetry. The students are devoted to medicine, but many are also trying to figure out partnering and parenting.

It's a hard switch, from the pursuit of a profession's goals to living your own life. All their schooling to this point has been work that brings you toward an accomplishment. Medical training is full of accomplishments—complete that course, pass that test, earn that degree, match in that residency, secure that fellowship—and medical students have been selected for their remarkable ability to accomplish. Students talk about how they mastered the four Ps—*performing, perfecting, pleasing, proving*—in order to get this far. They have two more schoolhouse accomplishments—selecting a specialty and matching at a teaching hospital—before medicine's dreams are realized.

What do you do after you realize your profession's dream?

The philosopher Kieran Setiya says that this question occurs for most of us in midlife. When you reach midlife, he observes, you look back at your travels, surveying the paths you took, the paths you did not take, and the paths you ruined. This can be distressing, as you realize that fewer choices are available to you at midlife. Some options have permanently expired, and there is no objective way to tell if you traveled the best path. And you can find yourself thinking unanswerable questions. *Was cardiology really the right field for me? Should I have skipped med school entirely? What would it have been like to be a poet? To have followed Virgil instead of Hippocrates?* When asking these midlife questions, you can become bored by past accomplishments but feel unable to set out toward radically new ones. Setiya's advice is to seek the value you receive from being immersed in the activity of daily life [114].

The paradox of a medical career is that medical training is about pursuing accomplishments, the hero work, but the actual practice of medicine is about caring for the sick. When you care for patients day in and day out, the value comes from being immersed, day after day, in the care of the people you meet as patients. It's not heroic, like in medical dramas, but endurance in the daily acts, much like the parenting and partnering decisions they are simultaneously making.

These days, the average student enters medical school just shy of twenty-five, graduates just shy of thirty, and completes training in their early to mid-thirties. Their prime years for the two other Ps—*partnering, parenting*—are spent in classrooms, call rooms, and clinical spaces.

And yet they partner. Physicians are more likely than most Americans to marry, as about four out of five physicians are married [115]. Dr. Adams met her own future husband in the summer after her first year of med school. Among med students, that summer has a certain poignancy—the last student summer and the last summer vacation until retirement—that makes it ripe for romance. Their spouses are likely to experience marital satisfaction as a function of how much time they spend with their physician spouse while awake. The more a physician works, the less likely it is that their spouse reports satisfaction [116]. Still, only about one in five physicians will divorce, which is a lower rate than other professionals, even lower than that for other health professionals [117]. Female physicians are more likely than male physicians to marry a physician. And some commentators observe that the kind of dual-physician marriage to which Mallory has said yes may be an advantage. After all, you are married to someone who understands the life [118, 119]. The price of that understanding is that being a physician married to a physician can mean less of the time together that typically leads to marital satisfaction.

And yet they parent. About four in five female physicians will have children, birthing on average 2.3 children, more than the average American woman's 1.9 children [120].

And yet they enter training programs designed to delay partnering and parenting. Osler himself married at the age of forty-two and counseled similar forbearance. For Osler, spouses and children were insignificant others to a true physician, because it was in the relationships with patients that a physician realized himself. The partners Osler prescribed were partners in medical practice. The parenting Osler practiced was teaching trainees. To trainees, Osler wrote, "What about the wife and babies, if you have them? Leave them! Heavy as are your responsibilities to those nearest and dearest, they are outweighed by the responsibilities to yourself, to the profession, and to the public" [36]. It's hard to imagine Osler carrying a breast pump and, as many female physicians do today, writing clinical notes while lactating in a hospital's call room. For Osler, being a physician was a way of life whose responsibilities outweighed familial responsibilities.

For the next century, a version of this counsel was given to medical students and enshrined in training structures. Teaching hospitals either prohibited or actively discouraged the appointment of married physicians to internships until the 1950s [121]. Teaching faculty encouraged engagement in medical labor over entanglements of the heart. The result was that American physicians were more likely to delay marriage and less likely to marry a peer than other professionals until the last decades of the twentieth century [20]. Even today, a female physician has, on average, her first pregnancy at age thirty, four years later than the average woman. One cost of starting later is that one in four female physicians experience infertility, twice the rate of the average American woman [120]. The demands of doctoring change a physician's family.

. . .

Mackenzie's musician husband keeps house so she can attend to the hospital's clinical demands.

"He's not in medicine, which has its own challenges, in terms of not being able to totally understand something that I'm going through. And I think it has some perks, in terms of he gets home from his job and can do the laundry. I think the benefit of him not being in medicine is that—this is going to sound terrible—I don't have to be there for him in the same way he has to be there for me. I don't have to worry about helping him through the same process as I'm going through. I can support him in other ways, but those are much easier ways than the way that he supports me." They have a deal: partnering now, with a division of labor. "There's the lack of true understanding, even though he really wants to understand, but he does everything in our house—dishes and laundry and groceries—and is very caring."

They have sketched out the next decade. They hope to parent after Mackenzie completes training in primary care and public health. Mackenzie wants dual training because structural problems like health inequity, racism, and social determinants of health have become even more pressing to her as she has accompanied patients—so pressing that next year she will take a leave of absence to pursue an MPH, delaying her final year of medical school by a year. The plan: complete an MPH now so that they can have kids during residency. For residency itself, Mackenzie is starting to think that it is time to leave her native state. Mackenzie is not yet sure where she wants to end up, but she leans toward a primary care program at an academic medical center.

As she awaits an application and interview process that will narrow her varied dreams into a single reality through the Match, Mackenzie finds that the clinical year narrows her intimate circle. "I've had to prioritize. I prioritize my family. I haven't missed any major family events the whole year." She let go of peripheral friendships. She held on to her significant others. Mackenzie is figuring out parenting and partnering, all while following an academic medicine model designed for the men who could follow Osler's counsel that partnering and parenting responsibilities "are outweighed by the responsibilities to yourself, to the profession, and to the public."

Halfway through the year, Maggie Kriz is learning how the responsibilities of hospital and home can bleed into each other. Maggie acts likes a physician, a physician with a lot of affect, a lot of presence. She speaks loudly, she cries often, and her laughter enlivens any room. It also keeps her close to her family, her fiancé's family, and the many people with whom they grew up, who are starting to rely on her in new ways. Her circle has not narrowed. Instead, her circle has begun to bring its medical questions to her.

"I recently had a family member who had gone on some new antidepressants and ended up being very manic. And it was very interesting because a lot of other people were like, 'She's acting a little weird but it seems like she's doing better than she was.' And I had to say, 'This is really bad, and she needs to be off of these medications, like, yesterday.'"

It was the kind of clinical one-liner Adams was looking for—good intentions, bad outcome. Maggie found it in her own family. Maggie knows and respects the rules about not doctoring your family. She encourages them to seek formal care, but she also feels herself becoming a medical authority for her family and friends. She feels it changing their relationship. She is learning what is serious and what is routine. She can tell her significant others whether to take their concerns to a doctor or whether their symptoms are normal, a skill her family and friends are relying on. They call her after visiting a physician. "My family members go to the doctor and when things aren't explained super explicitly to them, they ask me questions about what's going on. And then I explain to them what is happening."

What is happening to Maggie is all the changes.

Maggie had already been dating her old friend Sean—they met in middle school, traded notes in ninth-grade chemistry class, and adventured together in college—for a decade when he recently asked Maggie to marry him on the top of a 90-meter mountain bike jump in their hometown. Surrounded by their friends, decked out in Hawaiian shirts and brightly colored leggings, Maggie said yes. Maggie, like Mallory, will wed after the clinical year.

A June wedding, a mountain field, a friend's land. Dancing, drinking, and tacos to soak it all up. She's confident that it will be fun but knows she can't be the one to do the planning.

"I don't really care about flowers or colors, or whatever people worry about with weddings. I don't understand that. I just don't have the bandwidth. I was talking to my mom the other day because we're getting ready to send out our formal invitations. 'Mom, I need you to make my registry. I can't do it.' I don't have time to research the best knives and cutlery."

Her mother agreed to pick up the slack and pick out the utensils. Maggie's brother-in-law will photograph the festivities. Her stepfather will make the cake. Her aunt will arrange the flowers. They will make merry. And, eventually, there will be children. Her circle will keep expanding.

After seeing friends and family struggle to get pregnant in their late thirties, she is determined to start sooner. "We're probably going to start earlier and have kids during residency and just make it work. We can hopefully stay in Colorado so that our family can take care of our children for us. And luckily Sean is not in medicine, so he is much more flexible." Maggie is trying to marry and mother, all while doctoring. Both require presence, practice, and practical knowledge. Both teach you how to juggle multiple tasks. Both teach you to eat quickly while standing up. Both teach you to expect explosive bodily fluids at any time. Both teach you to prioritize other's needs above your own. Both teach you to party with the people who help you along the way.

· · ·

On the first Thursday after Thanksgiving, the students are in their classroom. Before they pass the chalice, Dr. Adams asks about the holiday. Most of the students stayed close, celebrating with family. Maggie went the farthest and the highest, ascending above 10,000 feet to ski her home mountain. She describes early season powder and the snow report. The report everyone is waiting to hear comes from Mallory. Over the holiday, her boyfriend asked Mallory to dress up for a cocktail party at a resort hotel in his hometown. Looking sharp, they were walking around its lake, when he stopped and stooped to one knee. He asked the question while a friend, previously hidden, snapped pictures of Mallory's answer. Her yes turned his nervousness into their shared joy.

Mallory beams as she passes around her phone. Her classmates clamor to see the pictures of the post-acceptance embraces. As the pictures circulate, her classmates produce a celebratory feast. Sarah Bardwell bought Ben and Jerry's ice cream from the 7-Eleven. Someone else bought Utz chips from the hospital's gift shop. Someone even made it to a grocery store for a precut fruit plate. And, of course, there is the traditional engagement gift: spicy jalapeno ranch popcorn. They open Martinelli's because real champagne will have to wait and chat about Mallory's wedding plans—she wants to marry within the year and enter the Couples Match.

Chapter 18

FORGETTING CURVE

ITZAM IS STARTING TO FEEL ready for his Match because his patients are calling him "Doctor." It's different from the traditional clinical year experience. Itzam talks to his classmates outside the LIC, the ones who try on different roles, one after another, by progressing sequentially from trying out being a neurologist for a couple of weeks, to being an obstetrician for a few more weeks, to abruptly spending a week as an anesthesiologist. These classmates never settle into a role, a place, or relationships. They tell Itzam they often have a new teaching physician every day and a new clinic or hospital every few weeks. They tell him that few people remember their name, so they often feel unnecessary to the clinical teams to which they are assigned. These classmates complain that they must turn away the underserved, uninsured, and undocumented patients whom Itzam can see. They must move on from patients quickly, so they end up remembering diseases more than patients.

Knowing patients well is what surprises Itzam the most. In the first half of his clinical year, he saw one patient for fifteen encounters. Itzam met her on the first day of internal medicine, and he was there when she went to specialists and surgeons, to clinics and operating rooms. At some point, she began calling him "Doctor." Earning the title from patients is part of the success Dr. Adams is seeking.

. . .

"Success is these students being interested in our patient population. Success is if they continue to serve them when they finish."

To a room full of already overworked physicians, Dr. Adams is explaining why they should precept, or teach in a clinical setting, an LIC student. These faculty already supervise regular med students, who follow along as the faculty see their patients for a few weeks or a month. If they volunteer to supervise an LIC student as well, these faculty will take on a med student for a year and the student will add additional patients to the faculty panel. The LIC students will mean extra work, and Adams has no extra pay to offer. Adams apologizes in advance, admitting that the extra work will manifest itself in every form of communication short of carrier pigeons. LIC students will engage them in group chats, forwarded emails, sticky notes, text pages, chart notices, and even the occasional outdated voice message. She admits that her students can be a bit much.

Some students make it a lot much. Those students add too many patients to a preceptor's already overfull clinic. She recalls a former student who kept identifying HIV-positive patients without a primary care physician and enrolling them in her clinic. The preceptors, most of whom are primary care physicians themselves, laugh nervously at the thought of more patients needing specialty care being assigned to nonspecialists.

Adams encourages them to turn a student's eagerness from disadvantage to advantage, because the students will rotate with the specialists as well. "I will tell a student, 'Ask the nephrologist why that patient was hospitalized!'" Adams knows that LIC students are uniquely able to connect a patient's various physicians because they have worked alongside all of them. The students can provide the context, the significant details that are often missing from the abstracted version of clinical encounters recorded in the EHR. The LIC students spend a whole year at one site, instead of a few weeks like Itzam's classmates in the traditional clinical year, which means they learn from the same faculty.

When Dr. Hirsh, the Harvard popularizer of the LIC, studied LIC faculty, he found that they both bear more responsibility for a student's training in the LIC model and reap greater rewards from watching a student's development [122]. Adams pitches these relationships: the faculty will truly know their LIC students and be known by them. She recruits faculty who are both technically excellent and capable of forming relationships. Then she prepares the faculty for the LIC way to teach. She explains how to set expectations early, to politely shush an overly talkative student, to assess clinical performances at regular intervals, and to grade students cumulatively.

Med students are the kind of people who always care about grades, and this year's grades influence which Match they can secure and the kind of physician they will become. In the typical clinical year, students will receive a grade at the end of each experience. A student who falters can extend their clinical year to repeat a subject—whether pediatrics or psychiatry—that they did not pass on their first attempt. In the LIC's integrated clinical year, a student cannot repeat a subject without repeating the year. In the LIC, the grades are received at the end of a year. Adams wants no end-of-year surprises, so LIC students receive provisional clinical grades throughout the year. To chart their progress against medical students across the country, they will take nine national examinations for core specialties like internal medicine and surgery, each of which lasts two hours and forty-five minutes. The national examinations are called shelf exams because they are made of multiple-choice questions that have been shelved from previous step exams. Students must pass every shelf exam, but the scores only account for a fifth of their final grade. Most of their grade is based on their clinical performance as assessed by the faculty. If a student is struggling academically, Adams asks the faculty for early warning. If a student is nearing failure, she asks for immediate notice. A student who falters in the summer can be quietly rerouted. A student who stays through August must be remediated.

The faculty physicians before her will provide the clinical grades, so Adams shows them a direct observation form. They will watch a student-patient encounter and, using the form, grade the student's performance. The form's length elicits more groans from the preceptors. Adams parries, acknowledging that it is impossible to watch a student perform a full encounter; she suggests staying in the room only long enough to develop three actionable comments because three is about as many comments as a student can remember.

To reinforce the lesson, Adams runs the preceptors through a two-hour workshop on how to assess students and provide feedback. The preceptors' anxiety decreases, but their talk reveals the different ways preceptors use evaluation forms. Some want to strictly enforce standards, like gymnastic judges. Adams encourages the preceptors to think of themselves as coaches instead, providing actionable feedback to help a student succeed. The desired result, she reminds them, is for students to take over the positions of the gathered faculty in caring for the underserved. Assign three actions, Adams says, but remember that one goal.

. . .

Itzam's patient is remembering him as her doctor, despite his protests.

"I kept telling her not to call me Doctor in front of doctors. I kept reminding her, 'Hey, I'm a student.' But she told me she was going to call me Doctor because she felt like I was more her doctor than a lot of doctors."

The patient recognized Itzam's ability, and now, after he helped deliver one of her grandchildren, Itzam is following three generations of her family.

During his labor and delivery immersion, he noticed a familiar last name on the census. He thought they might be a relative but feared asking would violate his patient's confidences, so he never asked. "But on my night shift, I saw the whole family again, waiting for the baby to be delivered. And they were like, 'Oh, what are you doing here?' So, I got to get to know them more by helping them deliver the baby."

Afterward, the family invited Itzam to dinner. He could not accept the meal—that was Adams's caution about boundaries in American medicine—but he accepted the closeness it implied, and the experience of being selected by a patient, of being trusted by a family, carried Itzam on through the year.

"It feels like these patients in some sense pick you. You want to follow everyone, but for some reason or another, one patient tends to match more with your schedule, tends to match more with your needs." He chose this patient, but by seeing her multiple times in multiple encounters, she chose Itzam as someone who was enhancing her care.

That mutual helping of student and patient is part of the success Adams is after, and, five years into her experimental curriculum, the successes are adding up.

When studying her version of the LIC, Adams found that faculty were more interested in teaching LIC students than teaching students in the traditional clinical year. Preceptors got to know the LIC students well enough that they could tailor their teaching to each student's needs. Instead of canned lectures on parasystole PVCs or parasympathetic responses, LIC preceptors reported teaching what each student needed. Instead of assessing knowledge, preceptors reported that they could ask questions to determine how a student thought, not just what they knew. Instead of assigning readings, preceptors said they provided actionable feedback. Instead of having students observe them in clinic, preceptors reported providing students with opportunities to practice clinical reasoning. Preceptors, in short, developed a true teaching relationship with the students [123].

Adams's students are documenting that patients like these relationships as well. In a published survey of patients seen by LIC students, Adams and her students found that patients were initially unsure of what to make of LIC students. The students would visit them in multiple clinical settings and at all hours. The patients were surprised because their physicians did not behave this way, but the patients eventually took the students' repeated presence as special. Patients reported that they appreciated how students helped them navigate the health system and facilitated communication between members of the patients' care teams. The students earned patients' trust by building alliances. The patients reported being more engaged with treatment, attending more appointments, and taking more of their prescribed medications, simply because they trusted the students more [78].

That, too, is success.

Adams knows that the clinical year is often the most professionally formative year for a physician. You become a physician through relationships with your patients, preceptors, and peers. If your preceptors are disinterested, your model for being a physician is an aloof technician. If your preceptors are empathetic, your model for being a physician is an engaged companion. Adams has LIC alumni across the country now, at medical centers from Baltimore to San Francisco. Most are still in training, but they are starting to show up in faculty jobs. They might forget much from their LIC year, but they remember Adams's vision of success, a career built on relationships with the indigent ill.

Assign three actions, remember one goal.

. . .

When something is remembered, it can endure in institutional medicine's memory, even if it comes from a student.

Medical students have long performed research, but some med student research changes science. In 1831, the second-year medical student Filippo Pacini discovered, with his naked eyes, previously unknown nerve endings; when you feel pressure and vibration today, it is through mechanoreceptors doctors call Pacinian corpuscles [124]. A few decades later, Joseph Lister, the father of antisepsis in surgery (think of him when you swish Listerine), made several discoveries about the pigment in the eye and the structure of muscle during medical school, despite experiencing a nervous breakdown [125]. In 1901, Florence Sabin published the best atlas to date of the brain stem, based on research during her own student years, in which she created a three-dimensional model of a newborn's brain stem [101]. In 1921, the twenty-two-year-old medical student Charles Best helped discover insulin, fulfilling a promise to better understand the diabetes that killed his aunt [126]. In the 1950s, medical student Lisa Steiner was the first to describe how RNA works, even if later researchers, all men, claimed the Nobel Prize for that knowledge [127].

Medical students have long undertaken expansive travel, but some travel opens new vistas for others as well. In 1865, Williams James began formulating pragmatism while traveling the Amazon during a med school interlude [128]. The middle-class Argentine Ernesto Guevara de la Serna rode motorcycles throughout South America to study leprosy during his med school years but was spurred to become a revolutionary doctor under the *nom de guerre* Che Guevara [129].

Medical students have long undertaken world-altering schemes, but some schemes alter the world. In 1879, Katharine Bushnell finished med school three years early to fight sex trafficking [130]. In 1943, Alexander Schmorell organized against the tyrannical, nationalist leader of his day, marking Munich walls with slogans like *Nieder mit Hitler*, as a member of the White Rose; he was guillotined by the Nazis in the very year he should have been receiving his diploma, earning martyrdom rather than a medical career [131]. In the 1980s, Paul Farmer spent most of a year in Haiti, while acing Harvard medical school, so he could found an international nonprofit that proved that you could treat infectious diseases even among the poorest people in the world [132].

And then there is the student who benefitted from Robert Graves's addition of the second hand to timepieces more than anyone. In 1954, after morning rounds at the hospital, the medical student Roger Bannister became the first person to run a mile in under four minutes, completing the feat in 3:59.4 [133]. Bannister later wrote, "There was a moment of mixed excitement and anguish when my mind took over. It raced well ahead of my body and drew me compellingly forward. There was no pain, only a great unity of movement and aim. Time seemed to stand still, or did not exist" [134]. Bannister's mind drew his body forward—as it does for all real medical students—into a new way of being in the world.

The question for Adams is whether her students' own contribution—not to research, travel, world-alerting schemes, or athletic feats but to a new way of becoming a physician—will similarly endure in medicine's memory.

. . .

Itzam experiences the new way as he builds a student's version of a practice. In his pediatrics encounters, he found himself being asked to become the physician to the children's parents. Then, when he saw the parents, he accompanied them across clinical sites. When patients became acutely ill, he was the one who understood what it would take for them to be healthy again.

"I think that's where my role becomes a little more valuable. There was one patient with a really crazy medical history. He decompensated at the clinic, and I was the one who took him to the ER. When all of the attending physicians met me, I realized, 'Oh, yeah, this is where I come in.' They started asking me which medications he took, what happened before, why he was there. I basically knew everything about this patient. In the ER, they do a bunch of tests, but they were able to remove some tests after I told them why he was hypertensive and all these things."

"He was super, super grateful for me to be there. But I don't think he knows how grateful I was for the opportunity that he gave me to play a role in his health care and learn." Itzam will remember.

. . .

What medical students remember and what they forget is a significant question for all medical schools. A good physician knows how much she forgot in order to remember the little she now knows. To help physicians remember only the crucial information, medical educators must understand how forgetting happens.

Forgetting happens, the German psychologist Hermann Ebbinghaus discovered, on a decaying curve. Around the same time that Osler was reformulating medical education, Ebbinghaus spent seven months teaching himself a row of thirteen nonsense syllables to the point that he could correctly recite the row twice. He measured the time it took to first learn the row. He repeatedly returned to the nonsense syllable row later—twenty minutes, one hour, nine hours, one day, two days, six days, and thirty-one days—and measured how much time it took to relearn the row. The difference between the times, Ebbinghaus concluded, was a savings of time spent between learning and relearning. He found that the learning savings eroded over time; it gradually took him longer to relearn what he once knew.

The distance from initial learning mattered, but other things mattered too.

The time of day mattered. Ebbinghaus tested himself at 10:00 a.m., noon, and 7:00 p.m.; he found that material learned in the morning had a higher savings rate. And learning was consolidated better if he got a good night of sleep after the first learning of a row.

The rhythm mattered. He preferred to recite in three-quarter time.

The pace mattered. He kept himself to 150 beats per minute.

With all of these findings, Ebbinghaus was able to determine the shape of forgetting: $x = [1 - (2/t)0.099]0.51$, where x equals 1 minus savings at time t (in minutes). [135].

Ebbinghaus showed that the first day after learning something is when the steepest memory loss occurs. If you cannot remember something the next day, do not bet on remembering it later. If you remember something a day later, you have a chance of remembering it a month later if you repeat it and review it. A memory strengthens and you flatten the forgetting curve.

The LIC fights the forgetting curve by reinforcing material repeatedly over time at a human rhythm and pace. The shape of remembering, the LIC argues, is a human relationship.

. . .

Pushing your mind ahead of your body, through excitement and anguish, until actions and facts are encoded in memory is one of the challenges of medical school. You must master so much, all while finding your Match in one of its medical specialties and subspecialties.

To remember so much, you must fight the forgetting curve, so that the information lives in memory.

Adams dreams of scaling up the LIC, to teach dozens of students. For now, Adams is fighting forgetting a few students at a time. Standing at the classroom whiteboard, Adams encourages the LIC students to select their opportunity from the chalice while they share snacks. They eat Skinny Pop popcorn, Halls sugar-free lemon cough drops, and Midnight Beauty grapes, while working through clinical cases on the various ways the lungs pop, sour, and expand. They happily spend the afternoon together, a master physician and the students she is training to replace her. The students speak openly, allowing their thinking to surface. Adams corrects them often, but in a way that encourages them to speak again. The tone, throughout all the hours of being together in one room with fluorescent lights and modest, crowded furnishings, remains warm and engaged. At the end, Adams will remark on how much fun she had, but for now she is back to pathophysiological explanations and memory aides and clinical pearls, like "Burn it into your brains. When you see schistocytes, think hemolytic anemia."

Burn it into your brains.

Fight the forgetting curve.

The shape of remembering is a relationship.

. . .

Itzam swears he will remember the lessons he is learning because he can see how they are changing how he relates to others.

"I feel like I have grown, not only in my knowledge but also in my personal development of how I talk to friends, how I understand people outside of medicine, how I interact with my family, my wife, my wife's family, my friends' families. I think medicine is not only a degree; the job is really a lifestyle change."

Itzam rattles off a list of all the things medicine teaches him about health, but his list quickly leads to how his newfound knowledge will improve the health of his wife, their future children, their family, and their friends. He is thinking relationally: Itzam mentors a high school student, visiting him a couple of times a month and taking him to visit local colleges, because part of being a physician, Itzam believes, is helping the next student in line.

Only part. Itzam knows that only a patient can recognize a true physician. The medical school will have its graduation, residencies will have their Match, but patients make you a true doctor. A few patients already appreciate how well Itzam hears and follows them, leading them to call him "Doctor." He appreciates the compliment, but he knows that it will take much more experience to become recognized by all his patients as a true physician. "I think I'm not going to become a doctor until 10 years after residency. I realize that it's one thing to know this disease has A, B, C, and D symptoms, and if you're diagnosed with this, then you treat it with this medication." It's another thing to see so many patients and know them so well that he can truly understand. When he can understand a patient's experience, not just the medical facts of a disease, Itzam says, "I feel like that's when it becomes real."

Chapter 19

FALLS RISK

OPENING AN EXAM ROOM DOOR, Mallory Myers finds her hollowed-out cowboy. Mateo is in his sixties but has the medical problems of a man decades older. His body mass index has plummeted to 12, a dangerously underweight territory where it is hard to stand, let alone walk. Mallory sees that his blue jeans have so much excess fabric that he needs his cinched-up brown leather belt, hand-tooled with Denver Broncos insignias, to keep them from falling onto his black boots. His belt buckle, bejeweled with four large costume jewelry rubies, tacks down his maroon western shirt and the black Henley shirt underneath it. His black leather jacket so completely drapes his frame that Mallory doesn't notice the fifteen pill bottles he carries in its pocket until he pulls them out, one at a time, stilling his tremulous left hand with his right hand. His brown eyes, set down in the deep watering pools of his sockets and framed by eyebrows that have not been fenced in for years, make constant eye contact. So long as he looks directly at Mallory, he can read her lips to compensate for his loss of hearing. He hands over various handouts about various illnesses from various doctors to Mallory.

Mallory organizes the disorganized papers into a story. He has appointments for cardiology and surgery but doesn't have a ride to attend them. He turned away Meals on Wheels because they served low-calorie, low-flavored food, never the green enchiladas he likes. He cooks for himself, but he struggles because of his eyesight, so the best he can usually do is canned beans. His best, the clinic's scale confirms, has him losing weight between each visit.

He was hospitalized the week before and is still wearing its plastic wristband. Hospitals encircle each patient's wrist with warnings—the medications that swell their throats shut, what actions to take if their heart stops beating, whether they are at risk of falling—printed on a plastic bracelet. For Mateo, the bracelet came too late. He had already suffered a fall that resulted from a failure of his body and community. The hospital stood him up with medications and fluids and rest. They scheduled a follow-up visit with Dr. Adams. At this point in the year, Mallory knows what Adams would do. Mallory listens to Mateo's heart and lungs, feels the pedal pulses on his emaciated ankles, and asks to see his feet. Mateo refuses. She pleads. Mateo stands firm in his refusal: no foot examination.

. . .

We pitch, plunge, stagger, stumble, topple over, tumble down, crash, come a cropper, lose our footing, lose our balance, keel, knock over, grabble, go down, and, like Mateo, trip up and take a header. For an old cowboy, falls increase the chance he will break a brittle bone or bleed within his brain. A fall, in its precise medical definition, is an unplanned descent to the ground, but in the life of a patient, it can be the dividing line between home and nursing home, between living in the community and being institutionalized. A fall means a different future, moving you ahead sooner to where you belong. Running is, after all, a controlled fall.

Some are running, some are shambling ahead, but all the students are now falling in with their futures, with what kind of physicians they will become.

Adams advertises the continuous relationships with the preceptors as formative, and in the class a year ahead of Mallory, Catherine Ard had that experience. She began the year thinking about psychiatry or obstetrics or even emergency medicine. In the hospital, she liked them all except internal medicine. It felt fractured, with new patients every day. But she found the continuity she craved in the internal medicine clinic with Dr. Adams and the patients they shared. Catherine will seek her Match with internal medicine.

"I love seeing patients time and time again. I love the complex, older adult that has a complex social situation and a complex medical situation." Catherine had found the challenge she had been looking for: a way to make the world a little better place, like she wanted to as an undergraduate; a way to build the kind of caring relationships she learned as a behavioral health tech; a way to teach; a way to be in the world. "I feel that internal medicine is really the place for me where I can make a difference and be challenged and be surrounded by wonderful, amazing colleagues and feel good at the end of the day."

Catherine found her place working with Adams, but many other students fall into place by working with the resident physicians. After all, the residents are just a few years older than the students—they are physicians like the faculty, but still establishing themselves like the students—so they speak in a way that resembles both the students' enthusiastic voices and the faculties' experienced voices.

When Mallory talks about her clinical experiences, she talks about how she falls in line with, or out of favor from, the residents on a clinical team. "I started out with internal medicine which was awesome. I had the nicest attending, the nicest residents. They didn't really expect a lot of work from me, but they taught me a ton." She thought her entire clinical year would be as good, but then the schedule shifted. She disliked gynecology—holding a retracting blade through hysterectomy after hysterectomy wore on her—but she liked obstetrics because she had a relatable resident. Residents had the power to make her fall in or out of interest with a specialty.

"My very last week of immersions was neurosurgery, and I had the most awful resident. He was borderline abusive to me. I talked with Dr. Adams about it. He was extremely tough on me, but not in a way that he was wanting me to learn, it was more like just finding little things to really berate me on. Made me cry in the OR. I will never, ever go into neurosurgery."

Mallory follows Adams instead. After ten minutes of kind entreaties with Mateo to remove his loose-fitting black boots, Mallory returns to the bullpen, where Adams is eating a one-handed lunch while writing a clinic note, and presents Mateo's clinical story. Adams interrupts only when Mallory gets to the moment of the foot exam refusal.

"It is not an option."

Mallory explains the persistence of Mateo's no, but Adams insists.

"On his last visit, I had him take off his boots and his nails were like concrete hooks. I don't think they had ever been cut. They were the craziest toenails I've ever seen. I went home and cut my son's toenails. He didn't want me too, but I was like, 'I've seen what can happen.' I worry about Mateo, and I've asked APS [adult protective services] and podiatry to see him."

Adams rises. Mallory follows. They head to Mateo's exam room.

...

Maggie Kriz sees the other side as well, the falling in with a specialty. Maggie is a first-generation college student, so she leans on Adams and her preceptors to guide her through career decisions and her future more and more as the year progresses.

Maggie cries tears of appreciation when she talks about her preceptors and how they truly know and trust her. She names other benefits of the LIC—iterative learning, dynamic scheduling, problem-based learning—but returns to relationships when she thinks about what her clinical year would have been like under the traditional model. The connection with patients is changing Maggie, but so are the connections with her preceptors. She started the year certain she would become an obstetrician, then she met Kenny and thought she would be an internist, but finally pediatrics changed her course.

"Kids just get really weird things that happen to them, like weird skin infections and very strange pathologies that you don't see very often. What I love about it is that they bounce back. I love that they're there for a day or two and they're really sick and they're on oxygen, and then they get better and walk out with a balloon. It's just such a magical place."

She met many magicians among the pediatric residents and fellows, but the master magician was her pediatrics preceptor, (no joke) Dr. Anne Frank. "She is just a very, very good teacher and an amazing woman. I'm actually planning on applying to med-peds now after learning about her career path and what you can do with med-peds." Frank trained in a residency that combined internal medicine and pediatrics, both three-year programs, into a rigorous four years. Maggie, seeing how the training shaped Frank, wants to follow. They are working together on a project to create a transitions-of-care clinic for kids transitioning out of the foster care system into adulthood. Maggie enthuses about the clinic, about building an alliance and then following a patient over time, potentially from cradle to grave, but also about the chance to continue her relationship with Frank.

"Dr. Frank has a way of making people feel really comfortable, especially teenagers. She has a way of making all kids feel comfortable. A lot of the kids that we see are foster care kids. It's incredible to see her interact with them." Kriz admiringly describes Frank's calm in dealing with kids going through the very hardest things. "I think she does it with such eloquence and grace and compassion." The tasks Maggie has been working on with Frank—seeing patients, talking about the future, helping with the foster care clinic—have deepened the bond between them.

To follow Frank into med-peds, she will need to secure one of the few spots offered each year by the nation's med-peds programs. Even a year out, Maggie has her sights set on one program, the University of Colorado's med-peds program. She wants to stay in Colorado; it is her and her fiancé's home, Frank is an assistant director of the residency, and the program's outpatient clinic is based at one of Denver Health's FQHCs. She already feels a bond with the program. Frank assures that she will be a great candidate, introduces her to other members of the med-peds faculty, and steers her to experiences that will increase her chance of acceptance, but Maggie worries. The program takes only four students out of more than seven hundred applicants; her newest goal requires passage through a narrow window during her next and final year.

The final year of medical school is typically composed of less demanding elective rotations and very demanding clinical experiences in the student's future specialty. The very demanding experiences are monthlong acting internships (AIs), where a student works on a teaching team under the intern's supervision while proving she can handle an intern's workload a year early. For Maggie, that means completing a rigorous final year while fitting in a wedding. She scheduled two AIs, a Step 2 exam, and a wedding between Memorial Day and Labor Day. Maggie is looking forward to a final year of stepping out around the state—rotating at the Children's Hospital and the University Hospital across town, marrying in her mountain hometown—until next spring, when she will match in a residency. She hopes it is here, so she can continue her work with Frank and with her patients.

"The biggest thing that I've taken from the LIC is the flexibility to make really amazing connections with people. I had a patient who recently died, and she was so wonderful." Sofia was only twenty-nine years old but already had alcoholic hepatitis, a disease that typically occurs after decades of drinking more alcohol than the liver can process. The liver becomes inflamed and stops working. The liver enlarges and becomes tender to the touch. The liver can no longer process bilirubin, so it enters the bloodstream and turns the skin a jaundiced yellow. The liver's failure eventually impairs the mind, leading to confusion, malaise, personality changes, even coma. It's a classic textbook-of-the-body disease, with a clear cause, a predictable pathophysiological outcome, and many targeted treatments. It's also a classic textbook-of-the-community disease, because such heavy alcohol use in a woman not yet thirty is a communal failure.

Maggie watched the failure in real time. Despite the physicians' efforts, Sofia died in the hospital. "It was horrible because she was just so like fun-loving and silly, and she joked around so much. As she continued to decompensate, I went and saw her in the hospital every day that she was there and, you know, even when . . ."

Maggie, tearing up at the thought of what she witnessed by being able to see Sofia daily, added, "And I think the flexibility in the LIC to tell your preceptors, 'I have a patient who's really sick in the hospital. I'm going to be late. I'm going to go see them. I'm gonna leave early to go see them.' It was incredible. She was totally encephalopathic. She looked at her gown and thought bugs were crawling all over her. But, you know, I would walk in, and she would know my name and say funny stuff like, 'Why are you still here? Go home. You've been here all day,' you know. When she finally died, it was really powerful because I had gotten to know her family. To walk in the room and her sister was laid over her body and have her sister just sob and say my name and be able to hug them and give them support through that. I think that other people just don't get the continuity and don't get to be that person for anyone. And it's interesting because I remember when I was driving to the hospital, when I got the phone call from the resident that she was going to be extubated to die, and I was driving over. I was just like, 'This fucking sucks. This is such bullshit.'"

Maggie appreciated that she could leave other obligations early or join them late so she could spend more time with the dying woman. Those bonds, formed over shared experiences, are the alliances that motivate students like Maggie.

"Because you care, you start to actually care about people and be invested in them getting better. But at the same time, it's one of the hardest things I've ever done but also one of the most valuable things I've ever done because you can be that person who is really seeing them through the worst moments of their lives and hold their hand and give them support. I have a letter from the family. I got a message that they sent a letter and it's over in the chief resident's office. I haven't picked it up yet. I'm kind of scared to read it. It's such an amazing thing to be there through the hardest moments in people's lives and it's really challenging but really rewarding. I became a doctor to be with people through the happy and the sad and support them and give them what I can of myself."

She is not naive. She sees the problems that previous generations have seen in our medical systems. But she has found alliances that work for her in the LIC. "Our health care system is not set up to give people what they really need. But I also think that you can express your compassion and empathy in a really small amount of time with really simple gestures."

. . .

Simple gestures of compassion build the students up, but they are simultaneously being broken down by the aversive experiences of medical training. In the words of the psychiatrist Robert Klitzman, "Medical training radically challenges these trainees, taking them apart psychologically, *wounding them*. They must put themselves back together, and end up identifying with fellow doctors" [109]. The residents and faculty a medical student encounters during their clinical year administer many of the wounds that make a student into a particular kind of physician.

Every year, the nation's twenty thousand graduating medical students are surveyed by the American Association of Medical Colleges. About two of every five graduating students who fill out the survey report having been personally mistreated during medical school, but fewer than one in four students reported it to a medical school faculty member or administrator. After all, faculty and residents were the people most likely to do the mistreating. More than half of graduating students cite the behavior of residents and faculty as a strong influence on the specialty they choose in the Match [136]. A related study specifically looked at the relationship between mistreatment and specialty choice. The most common source of mistreatment was resident physicians, surgery was the most common rotation during which mistreatment occurred, and mistreatment altered the specialty choices of students [137]. Resident physicians are closest in age and status to the students, and it is the wounds administered by those with whom you most identify that often leave the deepest marks.

Mallory preferred to focus on the positive but admitted that she could feel herself being taken apart and being put back together.

"I'll learn things during a session but then it'll be a week or two before I see that preceptor again, and I'm like, 'Oh, I'm starting from square one all over again.' It's really frustrating. I feel like I'm not making any progress."

She sought reassurance from her psychiatry preceptor, Dr. Elizabeth Lowdermilk. Psychiatrists are stereotyped as inscrutable sphinxes who listen without betraying emotions. Lowdermilk is more champion than sphinx, communicating emotions through expressive hands, head nods, and encouraging words. Lowdermilk reassured Mallory with an analogy.

"She said, 'You know, every LIC student goes through this. You're learning six different languages at once. It's slow at first but once you hit October, November, you're going to hit the ground running.' I was like, 'Okay, I'll hold on to that.' Then we had immersions, internal medicine immersions again, and I thought, 'I bet it's not going to be as good as last time this time around just because I had such a good experience.' But it was great again, and that's when I started to realize that I was making progress throughout the year. I've learned some things."

Lowdermilk was right. Mallory was getting the hang of it. But this learning still felt unsettlingly distinct from Mallory's other school experiences. She had been working toward perfection since high school, and she usually achieved it on exam after exam, but perfection was always out of reach in the hospital. Medical training was a different kind of experience, where you fall often and endure only if you learn to fall up. It was more like life than like school.

"You're going to make so many mistakes, there's so much you don't know. And so, something I've been doing lately is just being kinder to myself and allowing myself to struggle and remembering that I'm a student, and I'm not supposed to be perfect all the time. I'm still learning."

As she fell, Mallory was giving up the perfectionist ethos of her high-performing student years and adopting the *ancora, impara* motto of the lifelong learner. She took days off when she needed a rest. She saw a therapist for the first time. She learned to accept that she could make mistakes and learn from them. Still, she lost sleep over the anxiety that comes with the constant evaluation and critique that was reshaping her into an identity, the physician, that can never fully be achieved. You can always do more and do better.

Each time she presented a patient, Mallory found herself second-guessing her presentation and plan, trying to preempt a preceptor's negative evaluation. "I feel like I'm good at talking with patients and developing rapport with them, and that's something that has been pointed out on my evaluations. So, I feel pretty good about that. But what worries me is, 'Did I present this patient well? Did I include all the pertinent positives and negatives? Did I come to the right assessment and plan?' That's way harder for me, presenting a patient well, and presenting my plan, as opposed to talking with patients."

All year long, talking with patients helped Mallory fall back in love with the work. She could even feel that love with patients on surgery. She found it with Jalen on surgery.

"I met him during my trauma night call week. He was hit by a car, came in with intra-abdominal bleeding, a bunch of fractures. He was in bad shape. I was able to follow up with him later when he was in outpatient and when he went to the surgery clinic. I remember him being in a lot of pain. But I was able to help him figure out next steps, and he and his brother, who was also there, were really appreciative. And then I walked over with them to his urology appointment. I helped take out his stent that he had when he was in the hospital."

What stands out was how much it meant to Jalen that she cared enough to show up to his outpatient appointments and fill in the gaps in his memory of what happened at the hospital. "He asked, 'What did I look like? You know, how bad was I?' I was able to tell him what we did when he got there and how we stabilized him."

"I always feel really happy when I go see a patient and they've seen me several times and they're happy to see me again. And when the doctor that I'm seeing them with doesn't know them very well, I'm able to fill them in on the situation and tell them what's happened leading up to that referral."

Adams's gambit was working. Mallory still experienced moments of uncertainty, but she was making friends with time, even on surgery, by knowing her patients, her preceptors, and the whole system. Mallory was learning that the same patients were cared for on different services. She could see Jalen on surgery or medicine. What mattered was choosing how you wanted to relate to a patient like Jalen, what kind of physician you wanted to become through the Match.

"I know a lot of the people now. It's nice to feel comfortable where you are, whereas otherwise I'd be getting uprooted every month or so."

Mallory and the other students explain the specialties that they fall out of love with and fall into line with through stories they remember and stories they tell to explain their choices. Most of these students are choosing against surgery, but is that because of them, their preceptors, or surgery itself? Is it because surgery is the specialty closest to the textbook-of-the-body approach? Mallory says that the patriarchal culture of surgery has improved but that it still felt less welcoming than internal medicine.

"It still feels like this environment of 'My dad beat me, so I beat my kids.'"

It was peculiar. Mallory admires what surgeons do. She is now, for God's sake, engaged to marry a surgeon. She loves her future surgeon husband and even evinces love for the surgical faculty, yet she never tells them that one reason she would never select their specialty was her experience with the resident. Instead, Mallory, like most students who experience mistreatment, keeps her own counsel and allows one possible future to fall away. Surgery has fallen out of her future.

We all do this as our futures fall away. We have experiences. We draw distinctions between them. We tell some stories and forget others—all so we can fall into a single future.

"Everyone's so nice in internal medicine. The people that you work with really do influence what you're thinking about. I've seen that in my classmates too. My roommate had a wonderful experience in neurology, and now she wants to go into neurology. My boyfriend has an awesome surgery preceptor who lets him do so many cool things; she's really taken him under her wing, she takes him golfing. Of course, he wants to go into surgery, right?"

Mallory was, like the other students, falling forward through all the wounds of medical training and shortening her list to find her future, by seeing patients like Jalen and Mateo over and over again.

. . .

Adams speaks to Mateo in a determined version of Mallory's voice, but with the volume turned up. She kindly yells at Mateo to remove his shoes, and Mateo dutifully dislodges his cavernous boots. Adams begins documenting. Mallory presents at her normal volume. Adams repeats her words: same words, same tone, louder volume. Mallory looks like a younger Adams, with similar long brown hair and kind eyes. But while Mallory is well on her way to becoming a physician as skilled as Adams, Mateo responds to the difference experience makes.

As Adams examines his feet, markedly improved since his last visit, she teaches Mallory along the way. Mallory shows off the knowledge—of the body and the community—she has accrued since the year began. Together, they remove sutures, order labs, place a podiatry referral, explore options for home-delivered food and transit to medical appointments, and counsel the tottering Mateo to avoid riding his bicycle until his vision is fixed. Finally, Adams and Mallory promise to see him back in a month. They will both be here for Matteo.

Chapter 20

CONFIDENCE INTERVALS

*B*EING THERE FOR PATIENTS can get so messy that it messes you up. After working through their immersive experiences, following patients for several months in various settings, and learning with faculty physicians from many specialties, the students have encountered all the fluids. A single day on pediatrics where a student learned to always diaper a boy so that everything points down has unfolded into weeks of well-child visits where the students wiped off the whole rainbow of colored fluids spit up by children. Visits to the operating room have been made familiar by weekends inside its sterilized environs smelling the body's unsterile internal fluids. Nights on labor and delivery crescendoed with the broken dam rush of amniotic fluid and placental blood and feces that announce a new life. It changed the lives of the students. Now they know when to walk in the hospital and when to run. Now they know that they can do the work of doctoring. Now they know they will graduate. Now they need to select their specialty and its most likely fluid.

Most of the world recognizes a small number of accredited specialties. Canada has fewer than forty. In some countries, a medical student graduates as a general practitioner and chooses a specialty only after working as a primary care physician. In the United States, medical students begin their move into the nation's more than 160 accredited specialties—they run alphabetically from allergy to urology—and subspecialties in disciplines both common, like cardiology, and niche, like undersea and hyperbaric medicine, during their clinical year. While a physician can retrain—a cardiologist can make her way to becoming an undersea medicine specialist—most physicians practice in the specialty in which they signal their interest to the faculty.

Megan Kalata's signal takes the shape of a Valentine's Day card she and her sister make for Dr. Adams. It hangs on Adams's wall, in constant view, a flower print framing a pink rectangle of paper on which is glued a hand-drawn cartoon of a speculum and the sentiment, "Dr. Adams, you're spec-tacular, valentine!"

Megan is a maker, including valentines, cakes, and other kindnesses. She sends thank-you notes on paper shaped like piña coladas, riffing on her surname: *Piña Kalata*. She thanks others out loud. To herself, she silently sorts through her future—family medicine or obstetrics—and wonders how she can be certain of what kind of physician to become.

. . .

On a cool Thursday afternoon, Dr. Meg Tomcho begins with an open-ended question.

"How are your pediatric immersions going?"

Some students smile; others raise their thumbs. Tomcho, a tall, short-haired pediatrician who carries herself with the coiled energy of the college track athlete she once was and the studied caution of the introvert she has always been, waits a beat for further responses.

Megan gives it to her. "I love babies. They are so cute, and I love unwrapping them from their little burrito in the nursery and holding their hands."

The conversation opens up. Other students agree with Megan, but Mackenzie Garcia pops a grape into her mouth and says, "Yeah, but babies' hands are gooey and gross." Mackenzie's joke shifts the emotion of the room, and the students laugh but keep nibbling on their own gooey and gross snacks: bite-size brownies, berry-flavored Sour Patch Kids. Between bites, students swap stories of clinical experiences, in the same warm but professional tone that Tomcho established. Tomcho is both deeply engaged and deeply reserved, speaking with a careful cadence that invites reflection. She makes space for the students to chat, and they delight when they realize how their stories converge: one student was on the trauma team, assisting as they operated on a patient from an MVC, when some of the scrub techs and OR nurses were called out to a different OR, where another med student was working with the OB-GYN team on an obstetrical emergency.

Some stories happen in parallel. While those students were in operating rooms, Maggie was caring for an infant who had been born at home. Two hours later, the mother brought the baby to the hospital alive but distressed. Two hours after that, the pediatricians declared the infant dead. An hour after that, a nurse checked on the deceased baby, found faint vital signs, and called a pediatric code. The code team revived the baby, but the child had suffered an anoxic brain injury and this time was declared brain dead.

It is the kind of story that would cause most people to put down their lunches—a life whose first twelve hours consisted of birth, distress, death, revival, and then being born again into a life that resembles death—but the emotional tone of the room remains familiar and warm. They have become, at least emotionally, doctors already. They maintain the emotional distance to hear it as a medical story from which they learn rather than as a familial loss that they grieve. Doctors are people who hear horrors without choking on their lunches.

Tomcho certainly can, and she begins the hour's team-based learning assignment with the story of a sick child. Working together, Tomcho and the students weigh the available evidence for clues as to what is going on. They gather, organize, and discern what the signs, symptoms, and findings mean about the health of this abstracted child. After five minutes, Tomcho calls the students together and asks questions, seeking clinical answers and the reasoning behind them. When the students' reasoning is exhausted, Tomcho provides more information and sends the students back to the case to refine diagnostic possibilities.

After a few rounds of this, a student volunteer goes to the whiteboard to write a differential. Her peers ask about nuchal rigidity, petechiae, reflexes, and other signs of the pediatric body that might disclose the cause of the child's distress. She writes them on the board, then the students confidently work through each possibility, eliciting approving nods from Tomcho when they think like pediatricians. The case culminates, as the narrative work of a clinical encounter does, in the satisfaction of a treatment. Then Tomcho complicates everything by asking, "How sure are you that it will help the patient?"

Confidence intervals measure how sure a physician can be that a treatment helps. If Tomcho decides to, say, administer a measles vaccine, she might tell a parent that a single dose of the vaccine is 92 percent effective and that two doses of the vaccine are 95 percent effective. But when she is discussing treatment options with a student, she wants them to think in terms of confidence intervals. A single dose is 92 percent effective, but its 95 percent confidence interval ranges from 67 to 98 percent, meaning that a physician can be 95 percent certain that the vaccine will be effective for somewhere between 67 and 98 percent of the people who receive the vaccine, a wide range. A second dose increases the effectiveness to 95 percent and narrows the confidence interval to 82–98 percent. Two doses are the way to go if a physician wants more assurance that she can stop a measles outbreak [138].

Confidence intervals are the kind of thing physicians rarely talk about with patients because math often induces eye-glazing. Students must learn the math because confidence intervals provide a critical measure of how likely it is that a range of future outcomes will occur [139], so they have been embraced by medical journals and public health organizations [140]. Instead of a categorical answer—yes or no—about whether to administer a treatment, confidence intervals inform prudential judgments by giving a sense of the size and strength of results. There is more uncertainty in medicine—there are always a range of yeses and nos—than most people realize. Physicians are the kind of people who manage uncertainty by measuring uncertainty.

When a confidence interval includes zero, the range of outcomes includes the possibility that the treatment had no effect, preventing a physician from reaching any conclusions about whether the treatment benefits or harms a patient.

When a confidence interval is wide, the range of outcomes is variable, giving only some assurance that a treatment will have its desired effect.

When a confidence interval is narrow, the range of outcomes is precise, giving great assurance that a treatment will have its desired effect.

A student needs to know a confidence interval if they want to scale a single experience with a single person into multiple experiences with a population.

. . .

When Megan was a volunteer doula, she would ride the elevator to Denver Health's labor and delivery ward, imagining where her patient's mindset would be. Megan found herself thinking, *by the time I leave today on these elevators, someone's life will have completely changed.* When the elevator doors opened on labor and delivery, Megan would head to a patient's room and stay. If Megan labored with a woman enough, she could draw close and hold a woman's leg or talk in her ear as the delivery neared. She spoke in a language aimed toward the patient and her family. She learned how to make women comfortable through their labor. Physicians entered the labor room only infrequently and spoke in a different language, one not meant to be understood easily by the patient. *Complete. 90 percent effaced. +2 station. Give me a hook.* The physicians stayed in the room only for the drama of delivery.

Now Megan returns to the same labor and delivery ward as a medical student. She finds herself understanding, and even speaking, the foreign language of the physicians. "Who can I go do a mag check on or a labor check? Or who's moving towards delivery? Is there someone who's going to have a C section pretty soon who I should make sure that I meet and read up on their chart a little bit before we go back?" Instead of following one person through her labor, Megan now works at scale. Multiple patients, multiple rooms. She now knows more about the science of labor but laments that there is "not quite as much time to just sort of explore the dynamics and how people are doing individually." She finds herself thinking less about a woman's mindset and more about the numbers. "How many centimeters are they? How effaced are they? What station is the baby? It's all the numeric things as opposed to being a doula. It doesn't matter if your patient is eight centimeters or four centimeters because you're going to be with them no matter what."

"It's harder than I would think to keep people straight all the time and to keep what's going on with them straight, whereas for patients I was a doula for, I still remember individual things about them and their family members. I'm already seeing that when you're with multiple people, you're switching back and forth a lot more. Things get jumbled."

. . .

After Dr. Tomcho departs, an emergency medicine physician arrives for his Thursday afternoon teaching session. He strides to the whiteboard, erases everything, and tells the students they will work through altered mental status (AMS) cases from his clinical experience. He wears his experience on the ragged green scrubs that do not even bother to obscure his stained undershirt. The cuffs of his scrub pants are frayed and fall underneath the heel of his scuffed, matte black Dansko clogs.

"This case is from a few years ago, at a different hospital. EMS brought in a 26-year-old woman with AMS found alone. BP 200/100, HR 145, RR 30, Temp 40.5 (rectal). What do you want to know?"

As the students speak, he gradually fills the whiteboard with questions, guesses, and answers. The physical exam has three critical findings:

Neuro: 3+ reflexes at biceps, 4+ patellar reflexes

Skin: flushed, no rash, sweating

Abd: not gravid, mildly obese

Itzam Marin asks if EMS found pill bottles.

"Good question. Here is her med list." He scribbles out the following:

PNV w/ Fe

Diclox

Pepcid

Citalopram

Nortriptyline

The mix of abbreviations, brand names, and generic names—the language of the emergency medicine physician—is enough for the students to start thinking diagnostically.

"What is on your differential for this woman?"

The students think of overdose, meningitis, encephalitis, sepsis, substance withdrawal, seizure, rhabdomyolysis, and suicide. The emergency medicine physician writes each possibility but keeps prodding the students. They never add another common diagnosis, so he finally gives it up.

"What about thyroid storm?"

Itzam slaps his head for failing to see his own diagnosis in the patient's presentation. Then Itzam shakes his slapped head. "I want to quit medical school at this point."

The conversation ambles on, students and the physician taking turns asking questions and answering them. While discussing the Babinski reflex, an involuntary upward movement of an infant's big toe after a physician strokes the sole of the foot, the students debate the difference between adult and infant reflexes.

The emergency medicine physician laughs and digresses into a story from his own medical student clinical year.

"I was on pediatrics, and the resident told us to check the babies in the nursery for their reflexes. We needed to check their eyes for the red reflex, so they told us to take a baby and go in a closet to look. So, we each took a baby into the closet. We cradled their heads in our hands and shined our little penlights, but they would not open their eyes. We swung the babies up to our chests and then back down to induce them to open their eyes. As we did so, we cracked the babies' heads together, and they started to scream. We looked in their eyes and asked each other, 'Can you see it, can you see it?' The resident opened the closet and asked what was going on. It was awesome!"

Emergency medicine physicians love to swap stories that shock, especially when, in the end, nothing enduringly bad happens. The crying infants opened their eyes, the med students saw the red reflexes, and the borrowed infants were returned, with no documentable harm, to the nursery.

When visiting physicians tell their stories, watching how the students listen clues you in to the kinds of stories they will tell as physicians. Emergency medicine stories are about the drama of the crashing, cracking, and seeing the light. War stories. Mallory Myers and Mackenzie Garcia look a little put off because it is not the way they would make sense of the stories. They had both been listening intently to

Tomcho. When Tomcho told clinical stories, her patients sounded emotionally abstracted, like a collection of physical findings and lab values and imaging studies; pediatrics, like internal medicine, attracts the sober-minded, the statistically inclined, the students who care deeply but chart a story using data points.

The emergency medicine physician shares more war stories, both colorful and off-color.

A man jumped off a chairlift and suffered pelvic fractures, scrotal injuries, and pneumothorax. He came in as a trauma patient—so much to stabilize—but the question became why he jumped. "In walks this girl wearing fur-line boots and a fur-lined coat. I tell my resident he needs to go in there and get more information from his girlfriend. The resident goes in. When he returns, he says that she was not his girlfriend. The patient's from San Diego and they met on Tinder. He flew out the day before to meet her for the first time. They hopped on the first chairlift at a ski resort. He pulls out a ring and asks her to marry to him. When she says no, he jumps off the lift." The drama continues, and the emergency medicine physician must unmask the medical problem that caused such odd behavior. The story's end was the making of an unexpected diagnosis, an NMDA frontal lobe encephalitis—an acute infection of the part of the brain driving behavior and emotion—that drove the drama.

"I like to talk about Occam's razor and Occam's blender. In young people, it's Occam's razor, and you're looking for one diagnosis to explain the entire presentation. In old people, I call it Occam's blender; you often need multiple diagnoses to explain the entire presentation."

Explaining the entire presentation quickly—telling a clinical story so well it explains all the signs and symptoms with which a patient presents—takes confidence. The students find this physician's confidence brash. His stories are dramatic. His mnemonics are too, like what he calls the seven S's of car trauma. Sex is one of the seven, and he

tells about a woman who died after the man upon whom she was performing oral sex crashed his car. Many of the students cringe.

The emergency medicine physician soldiers on at the whiteboard, offering another case from another hospital, leading with the
lab results for a female patient. Her urine sample contained red blood
cells and proteins but no evidence of substance use. Her blood sample
was low on potassium and platelets but high on liver enzymes (suggesting liver damage), creatine kinase (indicating muscle damage), and
white blood cells (the kinds that are marshaled to fight off infections).
A qualitative human chorionic gonadotropin test was negative (suggesting no pregnancy).

The students suggest imaging; the physician nods. "We did that,
and while she was getting a head CT, she started seizing. How you do
sedate and intubate her? You want a short-acting agent so you can, after
stopping the seizures, get a mental status exam."

A student suggests an LP, or lumbar puncture, the insertion of a
needle into the subarachnoid space between the third and fourth
lumbar vertebrae in the lower spine. If you perform it right, you can
sample the fluid that surrounds the brain and spinal cord to assess for
signs of central nervous system disease.

"Yes, exactly," says the emergency medicine physician, "but
when I went to perform the LP, I found a hole in the precise place
where I wanted to perform an LP."

Confused, he waited. While waiting, a man walked into the
emergency department holding a three-week-old infant, asking for his
wife. The hole was the remnant of the epidural anesthesia the patient
underwent when delivering the infant.

Now the students are confident in the diagnosis: postpartum eclampsia, a complex condition that occurs when a postpartum woman
becomes dangerously hypertensive and spills protein into her urine. Un-
treated, she can seize and die. The treatment, though, is simple: give

magnesium. The physician did, and the patient resolved. Megan had the best instincts on this case. She suggested eclampsia at the beginning but was thrown off by the nongravid abdomen and the negative pregnancy test. She should have trusted her instincts. It was the kind of delivery story obstetricians like to tell.

. . .

On a recent night on OB-GYN, one of Megan's patients was sickened with preeclampsia, a related disorder of blood pressure during labor, and needed magnesium checks every two hours. "Every two hours I go in and ask her if she has any headaches or shortness of breath and right upper quadrant pain, and things like that. I could go in there and talk to her for 5 or 10 minutes about what she wanted to talk about, but I knew that when I went back to the team, they were going to have certain questions, 'How are her reflexes? And does she have headaches?'" Megan needed to know the woman medically and be able to speak to the medical team in her language. It was not a patient's colorful report of pain expressed in whatever idiom they preferred, but numerically rated pain localized to anatomy. She could do more with the bodies of her patients than she could as a doula, but at a greater personal distance. She had to employ her own empathy in less time, to earn trust as fast as a physician. The experience was helping her decide what kind of physician she will put herself forward as.

"I really like experiencing a little bit of everything and I love doing it through the LIC because I think we get a little bit more purpose with being able to follow patients and really care about people. And I'm still thinking OB or maybe family medicine. And, yeah, this year has confirmed that I really like women and women's health.

"I've had really great mentors in both areas, which makes it hard because I'm trying to figure out, 'Do I love the people that I've worked with, or do I really love the fields?' But part of the field is the people that you work with. My family medicine preceptor and I just really connected. She does a lot of women's health and runs group prenatal care which turns into group infant care for the same group of moms. That's a really cool model and incorporates what I love about women's health with family medicine. With OB, it's just being able to dig deeper and really work with patients who have complex situations."

Megan is weighing many factors: to care for women as a generalist or as a specialist, to spend a little or a lot of time in the operating room. She likes the OR more than she thought. She even thought about surgery. She likes being able to fix a problem, which is not the typical story a family physician tells.

"If I want to do something surgical, what I like about OB is that you still get to know your patients. Also, the surgeries aren't that long. I need to go to the bathroom and get a snack every couple of hours. C-sections are quick, they're great. I eat and I go to the bathroom. I've decided those are good things."

She is deciding against specialties without meal and bathroom breaks. No to surgery.

She is deciding against specialties that exhaust her. While she admires how emergency medicine physicians keep their fingers on the pulse of a community—they know when infectious diseases are waxing, when gun violence is waning—the work feels like emotional whiplash. "You go from hearing one person's life story and then you'll see another person. People are very vulnerable in the ED. I like talking to people and hearing their stories, but it's hard to move from one to the next so quickly." No to emergency medicine.

She is also deciding against the specialty that drew her to medicine in the first place.

"I came into med school really thinking I was going to do pediatrics. I realized that I love kids as little, tiny humans. I love holding the babies. But I have a problem. I like the idea of doing something more primary care driven where you get to work on prevention and bigger population things, but I don't love general pediatrics." She fears that if she becomes a pediatrician like Dr. Tomcho, she will be overwhelmed by the social determinants. "I like that you get to talk to kids about things like healthy eating and habits, and those things. But I know that you can't just tell a kid to go eat healthier foods. Maybe their family lives in a food desert. Maybe their parents don't make enough money. Maybe they are home alone most of the time and can't turn on the stove by themselves to cook something. I feel like I would get burned out by not actually being able to make those changes, like telling people over and over, 'Okay, here's how we can manage your asthma or prevent diabetes,' or things like that. But there's so many bigger changes—housing, food security, and health equity, and all those things—I think I would get discouraged by that." No to pediatrics.

Megan hopes to find a residency where she can combine her medical and public health degrees. She needs an actionable way to mediate between clinical care and public policy, between the body and the community.

She also wants a residency where she can form relationships like the LIC. Megan would stay here but suspects that it will not be an option. Some local residencies are loathe to interview candidates with a board failure, so Megan will likely leave to pursue her dream. As she anticipates her departure, she knows what she did not know at the beginning of the year: she will select the shape of her dream. She will have company as she does. Megan will soon select her future alongside her classmates, in the little room where they meet up every Thursday afternoon to share snack foods and speculum valentines, read the same materials, solve the same problems, dip their hands into the same shared chalice, and learn which specialties' stories they will tell.

Chapter 21
DAILY WORKS

$\mathcal{S}$ARAH BARDWELL TAKES the hospital's elevator up to the last stop, the ninth-floor nurses' station, to ask patients their final questions. Wearing her short white coat, stethoscope in its right pocket, Sarah signs into the EHR, which auto-welcomes her for resuming her epic journey and prints out the team's list. The single-spaced, 8-point-font, six-page list of actively dying patients is a physician's preview of the obit section. Sarah reviews the palliative care list until the team's attending physician, Dr. Phil Fung, a middle-aged man with the slim build and propulsive energy of a teenager still eager for what the future holds, arrives. Fung logs on, looking at lab values and perusing progress notes, occasionally slapping his close-cropped head when he hears of dangerous results or neglectful families. The team's nurse practitioner (NP) arrives and does her own review, minus the head slaps.

The NP's face, lit by her frequent smiles, is framed by brown hair so long that her ponytail falls down her white coat to the middle of her back. She is the constant on the service, another difference that Flexner never anticipated. Advanced practice providers, including NPs, physician assistants, nurse midwives, and more, have dramatically increased in the past quarter century. Some physicians see them as a threat. Others, like Fung, see them as essential team members. Physicians, like their medical students, rotate off and on, so the NP is the one who knows the patients best, and she helps them find value in their remaining days. It is the NP who tells the stories of each patient: who has declined precipitously but is still clinging to their past identity, who has reached their end and is readying to go, who is unable to either hold on or let go and so has family members competing to write different versions of their last days.

Around them, nurses dressed in blue scrubs perform the team's tasks. Nurses gather medications, answer phones, talk to families, arrange the staff schedule, and reset beeping bed alarms. Sarah does not know these patients or this clinical specialty, so she sits silently through rounds.

. . .

Sarah has been oscillating lately, between an encouraging feeling that she will become a doctor and a discouraging sense that she has wasted a decade. In the preclinical years, the shifts from the encouraging ramparts to the discouraging valleys usually arrived only on examination days. During the clinical year, she is assessed each time she evaluates a patient, presents to an attending physician, or answers a resident physician's questions. The intervals in which her confidence swings have been foreshortened.

Like most students, Sarah Bardwell finds that her confidence to tell doctor stories comes and goes with the feedback she receives. She forgets positive feedback. She remembers the negative feedback.

"I feel like shit all of the time. I'm not very good at internalizing positive feedback, so that is a real downer, because it doesn't come very often, and you have to cling to it." She shakes her pixie cut at her shaggy sense of inadequacy.

"I feel less and less confident that I will be a good doctor every day. And less and less confident that I can even do this job every day."

Somedays she thinks about dropping out. But she is ultimately determined to stay. Something about medicine, despite the ways it messes with her confidence, made sense when she started, and she wants to follow that sense to the end, wherever it leads her.

. . .

Fung interrupts the NP's summaries to engage Sarah.

"This patient is at the last stages of dementia. He is at the outer limit of life. You cannot communicate with him, right?" Fung pauses. Sarah nods. It is usually safest for a student to agree with the attending physician. Fung meant it as a rhetorical question. "Actually, you can, but it's hard. You can assess if they withdraw from pain, from pressure. If they eat. You can always be their doctor, always treat them as a person."

Sarah nods, signaling to Fung that she follows. The nod more than suffices as encouragement for Fung to keep teaching. An academic internist by day, Fung is working on a doctorate in ethics at night when he is not helping his children with their homework, and his teaching reveals a man who has been piling up ideas overnight, waiting to share them each morning. As Sarah listens, Fung moves rapidly between discussions of pathophysiology of delirium and dementia, the ways medicine has defined brain death over time, ethical theories about care and the end of life, and movies that dramatize these themes.

Fung wants Sarah to know not only how the processes work but also their limitations; as he says, "The process does not necessarily give you the right outcome, but it must be followed." He is mordantly funny about the perverse incentives of American medicine, reflecting, "If your goal is to cut health care costs, it's easy. Kill everyone over fifty. You will cut 85 percent of our health care costs and lose 100 percent of your humanity."

As Fung wraps up another stem-winder, Ed, the team's chaplain, arrives. Palliative care doctors treat people with life-limiting illnesses.

They emphasize care over cure, making them very different kinds of physicians. In their stories, the patient dies at the end. Their hope is for a story that is less about the physician's interventions and more about the patient's commitments. It matters, palliative care physicians say, how a person's story ends: is it a medical story of one procedure or pill after another, or a human story about how a person lived and to what purpose? Physicians have few answers about the purpose of life, about final things, so the team has Chaplain Ed to address what physicians cannot or will not.

Throughout the year, patients have brought existential questions to the students and faculty. *How could this happen? Why me? What becomes of me if I die?* Many patients bring their faith into clinical rooms, with medallions of the Buddha, T-shirts bearing a saint's visage, or prayer beads around their wrists. Most of the students and faculty do not engage these aspects of their patient's lives. Like smell, a sense of faith is neglected by today's medical training. Fung is different. Fung believes that physicians should follow patients into questions about final things. For Fung, it matters that the end of a patient's story is not medicine's story. It is part of his faith that there are stories beyond medicine's story. He wants the chaplain on the team so the team can engage existential questions and spiritual practices with the patients.

With the chaplain aboard, the team is ready to round. They divide the list: the NP takes the existing patients, Fung the new patients. Fung offers to take more; the NP demurs. Fung says, "I think they all need you. You know them better." The NP replies, "I think they all need Ed."

Fung turns to Sarah.

"Is there a patient from the list who sounds interesting to you? There are fifteen patients to see. If you pick one of mine, come with me. If you pick one of hers, go with her."

Fung was trained in the old way, where patients were simply assigned to students. He believes that Sarah will learn more by actively choosing a few patients. Sarah names a handful of patients who piqued her interest. She is initially interested in the younger patients but also expresses an interest in a profoundly demented man. The NP and Fung steer her toward this patient because his case is more medical and will give Fung more opportunities to teach. Sarah and Fung hail a downbound elevator. A phlebotomist is already in the elevator. She evidently knows Sarah and openly admires Sarah's haircut.

"Mmm. I have to get to your girl."

Sarah responds, "She does a good job," and gently touches a hand to her precisely cut brown hair, parted in a soft curl to the right.

"I've just got to stop going to little shops. I need to get to your girl. I love your hair."

Sarah has been at Denver Health long enough for the staff to see her. The phlebotomist offers no comment on Fung's monthly self-administered buzz cut—professional haircuts are part of what Fung gave up for doctoring. Fung knows the challenges of doctoring. His own wife is a physician who no longer practices. Fung sometimes thinks of quitting too, but seeing patients like these and teaching students like Sarah keep him in medicine.

After they arrive at the door of the patient's room, Fung resumes teaching.

"I give talks to med students. I ask them: What is the chief attribute of a good doctor? Last week, a student told me 'efficiency.' They said efficiency was the chief attribute! Not curiosity, intelligence, sacrifice. I shook my head. Look, efficiency matters. But it's not the number one thing."

To Sarah, the student's response seems earnest, an honest account of what it takes to be a physician today. "That's what I always hear from attendings: that I need to be more efficient."

"Think about that. When I was in training, we were asked to know *more*. To learn *more* science, write *more* papers, study *more*.

Now, medicine is all about producing quality metrics and physician billing and throughput."

Fung is concerned that the work of producing health outcomes is displacing the daily work of doctoring, of being present for patients. For Fung, medicine is an act of faith, a calling to the daily work of attending the sick. Fung believes that this is part of what's gone missing from medicine. He believes that physicians lack a sense of who they are working for and why. Fung thinks that it's part of why physicians are burned out. Physicians are so busy generating profit for themselves and their health systems, not to mention insurers and regulators and pharmaceutical companies, that they forget to encounter the patient before them as a fellow human being trying to answer their own questions of what they believe in and why. Fung wonders if the solution to burnout is to encounter the ill directly, especially the marginalized ill, and to teach others to do the same. Doctoring and teaching—for Fung, both are about giving away a little of yourself freely. That's how we flourish, Fung believes, by being in service for others. It's the part of being a physician that helps Fung when he experiences his own swings between being encouraged and discouraged by the physician's life. He usually attends on the general medicine wards as a hospitalist because it foregrounds the big questions of life. He also likes attending on palliative care because it foregrounds the biggest questions of all—about final things, about death, about faith.

After all, the progress notes atop palliative care bear a banner that warns patients: "Please be aware: this note may contain information about how long we think you have to live." The stakes in palliative care—life, death, and what comes after; matters of faith and what physicians offer to patients as they ask themselves questions. Sarah does not share Fung's faith but sympathizes with him that medicine should be offering something more, saying, "I want to do something different. I want to start my own clinic."

Fung sympathizes with Sarah's determination to find something better.

"I've done so many different things—worked in private practice, an urban Catholic clinic, and here for seven years. You have to pick your challenge. Every system has one. Ten years in, I've never earned as much as I did my first year in private practice. You take a 30 percent pay cut to enter academic medicine. I have six children and sometimes I wonder how I will pay for their school or for the care of my in-laws, but private practice was all about efficiency. Moving people through. I've chosen this instead."

They enter the room of an elderly white man with a neatly trimmed salt-and-pepper mustache on his face and an unkempt, retreating thatch of hair on his forehead. He is sleeping, naked, in his bed in a hospital built before Fung was born. Out the window, new high-rises are being birthed in the gentrifying neighborhood. In front of the window is a piece of poster board. At its center is a vertical 5×7 photograph of him smiling after a workout, gripping the towel around his neck at either end, looking hale. Around the photograph, the board is filled with signatures and kind words from well-wishers. It is a birthday card, from two years ago, from a different life.

Fung leans over the bed, gently taking the patient's hand and greeting him loudly. The patient opens his eyes but closes them again, unable to offer any more of the medical information Fung is after. Fung concludes, "You have to meet the patients where they are today." As they leave the room, Fung counsels Sarah, "No one knows that better than the nurses." They find the patient's nurse, who says the patient is no longer able to even swallow. Fung interprets, telling Sarah the best they can do today is avoid forced feedings. But then he reminds Sarah that they could do better, in a better version of health care. He tells Sarah about treatments like music therapy that he wished he could offer the patient, and then he catches himself and shakes his head.

"This is what it means to be a doctor. Most people could not walk in this room without becoming afraid. We enter the room, but we manage our fear by discussing pathophysiology and treatment options."

Fung intellectualizes in response to stress like most physicians, but he attends on the palliative care service because he sees this kind of medicine as a chance to encounter people, a place where you can help a person finish their own story well, rather than having it subsumed into one of medicine's war stories, a fight against disease at all costs—or worse, a fight against disease to maximize all costs.

Fung worries that the money American physicians make shapes them into something like the Puritans in Max Weber's *The Protestant Ethic and the Spirit of Capitalism*. Puritans followed Calvin. It is that Calvinist work ethic that informed Osler, Flexner, and the practice of every physician today. Weber's Puritans were enjoined to methodically and doggedly pursue their vocation, to take rational risks, develop innovative practices, and increase productivity. As they worked, believers were required to conduct themselves ascetically, abjuring the "the spontaneous enjoyment of life" [141, p. 167]. No seeking after pleasure, no acting on spontaneous impulses, none of the unscheduled time off that Bardwell craved. Believers disciplined themselves to use time to pursue rational goods. Sport was not play but a means to increase physical efficiency for work. School was not curiosity but a way to increase work productivity.

What Weber wrote about Puritans describes the culture of contemporary physicians—work constantly, increase productivity, seek innovation, and defer pleasure unless it can increase your work capacity. (The Venn diagram for the personality types of physicians and ultramarathoners overlaps.) To be sure, a physician should exercise, meditate, and sleep, but to increase the productivity of your labor. A physician can—and often should—skip traditional practices and familial obligations when work calls. When Weber wrote about how the Puritan way of life formed the blueprint for modern economic life, he implicitly describes how medicine became a rationalized version of charity: care for the sick became not a personal encounter but an exchange that secured a stable financial life. Efficiency is number one.

But Weber understood the trouble that ensued. Rationalizing the Puritan version of a calling enabled the development of capitalism, which then repaid the favor by devaluing the meaning of your calling into a *caput mortuum*, a worthless remains, a zombie version of a vocation [142]. A physician works like a believer, but without any of the old beliefs, and their world becomes, in Weber's resounding word, disenchanted [143].

In German it sounds frightening (*Die Enztauberung der Welt*), and in English it sounds clinical—the disenchantment of the world. In either language, Weber described where most physicians now stand. Physicians work like Puritans, but unlike Puritans, they no longer believe. Medicine has become ever more profitable because physicians work like true believers, but the profit undermines what physicians truly believe in. No longer seeking salvation through their work, physicians cannot remember what made the work enchanting in the first place. Some call physicians burned out. Maybe they are disenchanted.

And maybe, just maybe, physicians like Fung can bring back the old magic of medicine by teaching the next generation.

. . .

Over halfway through the clinical year, Sarah knows what she is looking for. She can see the differences between specialties, and now she is starting to see herself in those specialties. Sarah appreciates palliative care but is gravitating toward outpatient work. She likes the continuity, seeing the same patients over time in a clinic. She is thinking of pursuing a Match in the specialty most focused on outpatient work, family medicine.

"I really appreciate internal medicine. They look at all the problems, and it's a really in-depth, very linear thought process. I appreciate that. But it's very rigid and linear in the hospital—which makes sense. I prefer family medicine because it's typically not as rigid, and you're dealing with so many more factors outside of medicine. In the hospital, it's very 'We do this, then we get results, and then we do the next thing, and then we get more results.' In family medicine, you come up with a treatment plan, and then they go off and don't do it, and then they come back, and you have to figure out why they didn't do it. Did they not understand? Did they not like its side effects? Did they not have the money? There are so many other nonlinear, nonrigid factors to take into account in family medicine. It is about people, talking to people." Sarah wants to present patients with good choices, educate them, and see the benefits accrue over time. Daily work.

"I feel like my primary role is to give people information so they can make decisions about their lives that are based on things that they want to happen, as opposed to making decisions and not knowing what the consequences are going to be of those decisions."

Sarah is talking not only about her patients but also about herself. She is deciding her future, how she will put herself forward as a physician, the daily work she will take on and on and on, and the stories she will tell.

. . .

Fung asks Sarah if she wants to see another patient, a patient who is not on the printed list but is on Fung's mind.

"She's real, real nice, but real, real sick. She used to work for an international agency, lived all over the world. She started having chronic abdominal pain and was treated for infections, but it meant her diagnosis was delayed."

Metastatic abdominal cancer.

The patient is Sarah's age. While Sarah is choosing a medical specialty, the patient is choosing between palliative care and another bout of chemotherapy. Impossible choices. Fung has offered a simpler choice. The last time they met, he asked what she dreamed of eating. She answered with a Thai street food delicacy, so Fung called multiple restaurants in town until he found a cook able to make it for her as a special treat.

Sarah tells him, "That's nice."

Fung replies, "On some services, nice means compliant with medical treatment. On palliative care, you do not have to comply with treatment, but you have to engage. Nice means the conversation can flow. It means there is conflict, but the conflict can be engaged. Sometimes on palliative care, the conflict cannot be engaged, only defused. You have family meetings where everyone is yelling at each other. This lady is nice, so we can have the conversation about whether or not to engage palliative care."

Fung and Sarah enter the room. The patient is wearing black leggings, a flowing black top. She has blush and eyeliner on her face, AirPods in her ears. She looks like the professional she is but talks like a patient. "I need to stand for the conversation, because it hurts to sit down because of the bloating." She remembers Fung even though she hasn't seen him in a few months. They stand next to each other, with Sarah to the side of their conversation and a step back.

"I've heard you've been thinking about palliative care."

"I was, but Dr. __ thinks there is a real chance with the new treatment. If I can get my symptoms under control, I'll do those treatments."

"Okay. I just wanted you to know it is available." He reminds her of the offer to have the Thai food made for her. She thanks him but declines, blaming the bloating.

"I need to try some shredded pork first before I'm ready."

From food, the conversation turns flavorless, to meds and treatment options. *Phenergan. Lidocaine. Stents.* Sarah listens patiently.

The patient's mother arrives, takes off her winter coat, and puts down her bag. She listens too as Fung wraps up. He tells the patient that while he is not on palliative care tomorrow, he will swing by and see her anyway. Without warning or request, the patient hugs him, appreciating his efforts to doctor differently by being present, by attending whenever he can.

And then Fung and Sarah continue their rounds, examining patients and talking along the way, coming close to the deathly ill and turning the experiences into pathophysiological discussions, hairstyle compliments, favorite Thai food treats, and spontaneous hugs. Doctoring.

Chapter 22

GIVEAWAYS

TZAM MARIN PRESENTS a chalice exercise that will decide his own future. The case itself is simple. He sits while Sarah Bardwell reads it aloud.

26 yo Hispanic F with no significant PMH presents to IM clinic with CC of nausea, vomiting, dizziness. The patient endorsed mild episodic HA lasting 1-2 hours, no focal neuro findings. HA improves with rest and Tylenol. She endorses increased sleep, mild constipation. LMP in November. VS: BP 92/60, HR 92, otherwise normal. BHCG +.

Bardwell translates it in her mind. A young woman with no chronic medical problems presented to an internal medicine clinic feeling sick. Her headache improved with simple treatments. Her last menstrual period was a few months ago. Her vital signs are okay. A home pregnancy test was positive.

Itzam advances his presentation. Three images fill the screen. Bardwell and the other students recognize the shadows of the ultrasound stills. The shapes mean a baby, but Sarah sits still with the rest of the room. The case's first answer is a giveaway: the patient is pregnant.

Sarah whispers, "Whose baby?," immediately turning to the case's second answer.

Maggie Kriz says, "Oh my God, is someone pregnant?"

The students turn to Dr. Adams and ask, "Are you pregnant?" Adams shakes them off with nervous laughter. She has school-age twins at home and is not looking to raise infants again. She points to Itzam. The students cheer. Maggie pumps her arms in the air like celebratory lightning, which raises her out of her chair, and she races over to Itzam to hug him from behind.

"Oh my God, you're going to be a dad. You're going to be a dad!"

Osler's advice was to defer partnering and parenting until after you become a physician, but Itzam and his wife, Andrea, could not wait. Itzam will become a parent as he becomes a physician, dividing his time and giving it away to hospital and home simultaneously.

...

Osler was rarely pictured as a family man, but rather as a kind of solitary medical saint. In his most memorable portrayal, a drawing from 1896, Osler is depicted as a mustachioed, balding cherub in a garment that amalgamates a physician's white coat and the robe of a singer in the heavenly choir. Osler rides a purifying whirlwind into the clouds above the Johns Hopkins Hospital. Osler is held aloft by angel wings sprouting from his scapulae. A halo glows above his head as he gazes determinedly into the future, above it all. On the ground below him, infectious diseases flee. The drawing is entitled, simply, "The Saint" [144].

The image misleads. Osler was knighted but never sainted, and Sir William Osler never made any basic science breakthroughs or clinical advances against disease, infectious or otherwise.

What Osler did was create the social structures of a physician's life. He reoriented medical education around bedside teaching. He designed the first residency system for physicians. He helped build internal medicine as its own specialty. In each instance, Osler designed medical school, residency, and practice around a rigorous, self-sacrificing professionalism based at research universities. Osler called the resulting work a physician's "noble calling," like the labors of a knight, or the efforts of a hero. For Osler, this meritocratic work was a physician's identity.

Osler was a minister's son. He never so much lost his childhood faith as transferred it from the church to the hospital, testifying often to medical students, resident physicians, and practicing physicians about how being a physician was the calling around which a physician organized his life. To the places where he could not travel, Osler's sermons on self-sacrifice circulated in his absence. For two generations, every graduating American medical student received a collection of Osler's talks from Eli Lilly when they graduated, like a divinity student might receive a volume of scripture [145]. Osler's *Aequanimitas* was an extended hymn to equanimity, the even-keeled emotional composure that admits no disturbance when exposed to disturbing phenomena.

Much has changed since Osler. His ethic focused on the problems of the acutely hospitalized ill. Those hospitals were often a single building. The physicians who worked in them were often paid like teachers. The industry of health care was chores at the bedside of the ill. After the *Flexner Report*, the federal government passed out generative funding to the schools Flexner favored, including billions of dollars to support research from the National Institutes of Health and trillions of dollars to support clinical care through Medicare. The medical schools based at research universities grew large and lucrative until they dominated their universities themselves. When the foremost historian of medical education, Kenneth Ludmerer, ran the numbers at the end of the twentieth century, he found that medical schools' annual budget swelled from about $100,000 in 1910, to $1,000,000 in 1940, to $20,000,000 in 1960, to $200,000,000 in 1990. As their budgets grew, Ludmerer wrote, their social role shifted. Before World War I, they focused on education, training the best physicians to ensure the best health for the American public. After World War I, they focused on research, advancing medical knowledge to produce breakthrough treatments. After World War II, they focused on providing the most technically advanced care [86].

As the social pact shifted from education to research to technical care, medical schools expanded first into academic medical centers that dominated their universities, then into hospitals that dominated their town, and then into health systems that dominated regions. Today's health systems are regional networks of clinical care—with primary care clinics sending commercially insured patients to citadels of specialists for complex treatments—that conduct research to understand how better to deliver this care. Many have added another zero to their budget.

Today, what brings people to physicians are the chronic illnesses and even more chronic health disparities that sicken them. Hospitals have become profitable health systems that span regions. Becoming a physician has become the most reliable way to join the 1 percent. The health care industry amounts to $4.6 trillion annually. And yet medical education, training, and practice have, for the past one hundred years, remained variations on Osler's themes, where the physician is, if not a soaring saint like Osler, then his kind of noble medical hero.

Itzam is not looking to become a hero. He has decided that becoming a parent will focus his practice. He knows that becoming a parent will change him, but he knows that becoming a physician will too. He is here for those changes. He will be purposeful in the clinic and the hospital so he can be home. He wants to be *there*. And *there* means the home and the hospital. Itzam may miss out on some of the ribbons and plaques and awards medicine gives out, but his illness made it clear what mattered. He will partner and parent while becoming a physician. He will give his life away to home and hospital simultaneously. He wonders if it will be a better burnout cure. Health care says you beat burnout with life hacks, mindfulness techniques, or retirement planning. Those are all ways to organize your life against the wounds of medical training and practice. They can make you feel okay. Itzam wonders if the only way to feel better than okay is to give your life away to someone else.

...

The LIC students are all looking to give their life away but are not quite sure how. As Dr. Fung reminded Sarah, medicine no longer asks in the ways it used to, even though today's students are at least as idealistic as students from previous generations, so the students are looking on their own. Itzam finds it in having a baby while pursuing his grandfather's dream. Maggie Kriz and Mallory Myers find it in getting married while becoming physicians like their preceptors. Megan Kalata pursues a way to combine public health and clinical medicine. Mackenzie Garcia stays married while pursuing medicine as a kind of social justice. Sarah also wants to believe that medicine can be a form of social justice, but the clinical year has left her wondering if medicine is really about justice.

Three-quarters of the way through her clinical year, Sarah's medical knowledge has increased, but so has her concern about how medical training is changing her. With so much to see and learn, Sarah feels herself choosing between education and health.

"I prioritize sleep over seeing twice as many patients. Quality of life is a huge deal to me. And students say, 'This is why I like Dr. Adams,' because she cares about our life. But Dr. Adams says to us, 'You're really going to have to get used to getting to the gym, because this is the rest of your life.'"

Adams prepares students for the self-disciplining strategies a contemporary physician must undertake, and Sarah is reluctant to give herself over to the program, to accept that these disciplines will be the rest of her life. "It's just not. You can choose to work eighty hours a week, and be the director of a thing, and a manager of another thing, and a person on a committee and all this stuff. I'm not going to do that. I want to have dinner with my family. I'm not going to do this job for another forty years working eighty hours a week."

"I say 'quality of life.' Really what I mean is time off. That's what I'm actually talking about. Full nights of sleep, nights when I come home and I just don't do anything at all except hang out with my partner or, you know, *socialize*."

Sarah resists how the magic of medicine has been worn away by the labor of health care.

"I just hope I can find joy in this. I'm in such an adversarial relationship with medicine and medical school at this point that sometimes I'm just, like, fuck it. I hope that I can find a profession in medicine that I feel valued in and that I enjoy. That I am not so bogged down by the number of hours I have to spend on it that I don't want to do my work anymore."

Like Sarah, the faculty often wonder what it will take for physicians to feel good again, to no longer experience the work as dully discouraging. They wonder if physicians err by describing medicine as a noble calling while pursuing it in today's unprincipled health care industry. Are physicians giving their lives away to their patients or to an industry? Is a sense of calling being weaponized by health care? It leaves many physicians worried that there is a fundamental mismatch between what medicine and hospitals were founded to do and what health care systems do today. Today's health care systems want profit from a physician's calling and from hospitals, but the calling and those hospitals were designed to pursue an altruism that is more like Dr. Fung's prescription for burnout, direct encounters with those in need. After all, as Fung reminds students, the hospital is a structure developed to encounter the divine only through direct charitable encounters with the indigent ill.

The hospital was a revolution in altruism; the Greco-Roman world had no such vision of charity. They had hospitality because everyone eventually must rely on the kindness of strangers and because you never knew when you were meeting a god in disguise. But any philanthropy was directed toward the people you recognized as your own—family, guests—so you could earn honor and prestige. And the gods? Greco-Roman divinities were more likely to become swans so they could seduce mortals than to favor the poor. Greco-Roman philosophers rarely counseled students to address the fate of the poor, and neither did Greco-Roman medicine. If you could fly above a Greco-Roman city, you could see that the social structures of its altruism were baths, governmental basilicas, and public theaters—public spaces for endowed citizens rather than for a society's poor.

Cities changed under the influence of texts like the radical writings of Ben Sira. Ben Sira counseled his readers to give alms to the indigent and even to *lose* money on behalf of the poor because the poor person was their conduit to the divine, and the communities that accepted his challenge began building institutions to care for and encounter the poor. By the medieval era, if you took that same aerial view of a city, it would reveal that the social structures of charity were now public hospices, orphanages, and soup kitchens for the poor. What distinguished these charities was that their social shape was personal, requiring encounter with the poor [146].

Chief among these structures was the public hospital, a tradition inaugurated by Basil of Caesarea, the fourth-century polymath who also founded one of the first public health systems. Basil's hospital welcomed all, irrespective of their ability to pay, and was built to welcome strangers and immigrants instead of citizens. Altruism was for the benefit of the poor rather than the honor of the philanthropist. Poverty was not an abstract problem to be solved but a condition of people who were to be encountered. Money was not for storing up but for enabling those encounters. Basil gave away his own inheritance and called on his congregants to similarly undertake sacrificial almsgiving for the poor. His idea spread, endowing towns around the world with public hospitals. These public hospitals were structured by Basil's radical version of charity: direct encounter with the poor, at personal cost to the giver, as an encounter with the divine [147].

Denver Health exists because of Basil's radical charity, but it hardly dominates the city.

An aerial view of Denver, like most American cities, includes remarkable public spaces, such as parks, libraries, and theaters, but it is dominated by privatized spaces—football stadiums, luxury condos, and, tragically, most of its hospitals. Almsgiving is rarely commerce with the divine. Charity is rarely a direct encounter with the poor. Altruism is, instead, more commonly a charitable gala, an endowed chair, a named building, or a subsidized doctor's visit.

After their training years, few practicing American physicians can describe their work as Basil's kind of charity. Even if a physician lives below their means, their means are likely well beyond their needs. Their means would astound many of the people they meet as patients. If physicians work with marginalized patients during the day, most still go home at night to a life so different from the lives of their patients that it can feel as far away as the medieval world feels from the contemporary world. American physicians practice a professional charity that is more compound interest and defined contributions than radical charity. American physicians deduct their charity against their expenses, instead of their sins.

In the competitive world of medicine, where every action should be to advance your medical career, even parenting is a countercultural act. When Itzam and Andrea decide to parent during medical school, it's a small reminder to the students of what an enchanted version of charity looks like. A direct encounter. A sacrificial gift. Itzam and his wife Andrea would welcome a child, despite the constant labor of medical school, despite his own illness, and would care daily for a little human at home while he cared for adult humans at the hospital while earning a resident's stipend so modest it can barely cover most living expenses, let alone childcare.

. . .

Most physicians have adopted the Puritan reticence to speak about money. Sarah cannot stop talking about money. She is pushing back against the transformation of medicine's sacred duties into mundane chores for the vulgar health care industry, which is far better at promoting wealth for physicians and health care executives than the health of its patients [148]. She is pushing back on the Puritan work ethic and the capital it accumulates.

Sarah knows that the escalating expenses of the medical dream are, at present, too costly for all involved. She has heard faculty speak of their training days as a kind of initiation rite, like those for shamans and healers in indigenous cultures. Before duty hours restricted a trainee's time in the hospital, they worked constantly and were so exhausted that they sometimes hallucinated words and images. They experienced the hospital as a sort of wilderness where they became a kind of biomedical shaman. It was a full initiation rite into medicine as a kind of magic. That training was a kind of enchantment, they tell trainees. They suspect that part of why today's trainees suffer from burnout is because they have never experienced a full initiation rite, but rather a low-grade constant wounding. Today's medical education too often harms trainees without building them up, failing to provide the kind of transformative experience that summons up the old magic.

Sarah is not sure about all of that but agrees that physicians have lost the old dream of medicine, the one where they thought that it was a calling, a vocation. Now the grinding, repetitive work is disenchanting.

Sarah wants no part of a rationalized Puritan calling, of disenchanting work, of becoming a robot, from the Czech word *robota*, meaning "forced labor."

She wants a better dream, a new enchantment, governed by justice and mercy, community and love, so physicians can see the people they meet as patients in personal encounters, as Basil wished. He built the first public hospital on the outskirts of his town to welcome fellow travelers instead of settled citizens, irrespective of their ability to pay, in a structure providing the best medicine of the day. The best medicine of our own day is more effective and more alienating, the provision of medical care as a financial transaction. It is hard to truly encounter and accompany someone when you head home to a different life, when you define your contribution as a professional service for a professional fee that benefits a health system as much as (or more than) a patient. Sarah wants something beyond a faithless version of the Puritan ethic.

Sarah is attempting to maintain what makes medicine magical while managing medicine's money. She worries that the LIC was a relational interlude within the transactional symphony of contemporary health care. Patients and preceptors and classmates care about her, but it is only for a time. Sarah dreams of a structure that will allow physicians to recapture some of the old medical magic, Weber's *Verzauberung*, over the whole of a doctor's life.

Chapter 23

NATURAL ATTORNEYS

*M*ACKENZIE GARCIA IS LEARNING that you head home to understand the hospital.

"There are lots of patients that I've had a good connection with or a
lot of good follow-up visits and been able to be there as their physician.
My favorite thing is when a patient is starting to make changes. I like
being there when somebody decides they want to quit alcohol or decides that they want to work on weight loss. I've been involved in a lot
of moments like that, which I really love." The moments she loves
most are with Thurline, one of the patients she visited at home. "I got
to see her home, and there was a lot more personal connection there.
She was the first patient I thought of as *my patient*. And then it came
full circle for me this year."

Like all the students, Mackenzie followed a few patients closely
enough that the patients invited them into their own homes, where she
could see how patients arranged their space, how they stuck themselves in the world, and how home affected health.

. . .

In a way, Mackenzie was following the footsteps of an almost forgotten
pioneering physician, about whom it was once written, "She arrived
here in Denver some fifty years ago, a[n] excitingly alive young person.
Out to Crusade for the improvement of human relations."

The excitingly alive young person was Dr. Justina Ford, but the description was from her obituary, which hailed Dr. Ford as the "very first woman physician of Color in Denver and in Colorado" [149].

The future Dr. Ford was born in 1871, the same year as the future Dr. Florence Sabin, but they traveled different paths to Denver Health. Sabin went to elite schools, studied basic sciences, trained at the country's leading residency, and then took faculty positions. She encountered profound discrimination as a female physician but was able to use the meritocracy to break into medicine. She did it by beating male physicians at their own game, studying the textbook of the body so well that she published atlases of the brain and, later in life, learning the textbook of the community by leading public health efforts.

Ford, the seventh child of a mother who had risen out of slavery to become a practical nurse and a father who was also likely born in slavery, received a working-class education, earned her career as a community physician, left behind no publications, and spent her entire life knocking on the doors of institutional medicine, seeking the recognition her excellence warranted.

Straight out of high school, Ford studied at Hering Medical School, a coeducational homeopathic school in Chicago that opened before the turn of the century and closed soon after Flexner's report. Ford graduated in one of its first classes and made her way, in 1902, to Denver's Five Points neighborhood, just north of downtown, a neighborhood of immigrants where the frontier city's medical institutions rarely extended their care.

She paid the state $5 for a medical license, no. 3800, which allowed her to practice [150]. The licenses are issued sequentially, so the state licensed 3,799 physicians before it licensed its first Black woman. The professional societies extended even less welcome. The Colorado Medical Society refused Ford membership, which precluded membership in the American Medical Association and disqualified her from admit-

ting privileges at most of the city's hospitals. She practiced in the community. She tended wounds, nursed fevers, and delivered babies. Her
patients were the indigent, the immigrant, and the working poor. At a
time when most of the city's hospitals would not admit these patients,
just as they would not admit her to their staff, Ford remembered that she
cared for people in their homes.

They paid, but sometimes in barter: blankets, chickens, and
groceries.

They paid, but sometimes late: "There was one lady who couldn't
pay for her baby until the baby was thirteen years old. I'd forgotten
about that bill. But she hadn't."

They paid, but sometimes in loyalty: "I remember delivering a
Spanish mother when she was very young . . . thirteen or so. Neither
she nor the family had any money to pay me. The girl moved away to
California, and I never thought any more about the matter. But when
she was pregnant again, you know what she did? She came clear back
to me. She wouldn't let anyone handle her but me. That's the kind of
thing that makes a doctor proud" [151, 44].

Everything about Ford's work is the kind of thing that makes a
doctor proud. She saw patients from all walks of life. She provided the
best care she could. She worked tirelessly. "I get around the problem of
hours fairly well. I just get along without sleep when I must. I can go
two days without sleep. I've done it often. The trick is not to slow down.
Once I slow my pace I've got to turn in" [151, 43].

. . .

For Mackenzie and many of the other students, the best way for medicine to recapture its magic is to fight against social injustices just as
much as biological diseases. Before medical school, all the students engaged in some form of activism or community service. They found it at
least as critical preparation as shadowing a physician or participating
in medical research. They surely believed that clinical sciences and

basic sciences were essential to medicine, but what most of them felt were the stinging inequalities caused by the social determinants of health.

When the faculty wanted to assure them that physicians could address social determinants in each patient and even on a population basis, they cited Dr. Paul Farmer, the leading social medicine physician of his generation. Farmer thought of medicine as a personal encounter between a physician and their patients, especially marginalized patients, that extended the life-extending advances of modern medicine to people living in the world's poorest places. When he wrote about the work, he sounded like Dr. Fung up on the palliative care team, writing that since illness preferentially visited the poor, physicians should preferentially serve the poor. Farmer prescribed the corporeal works of mercy: *Feed the hungry. Give drink to the thirsty. Clothe the naked. Shelter the homeless. Visit the sick. Visit the prisoners. Bury the dead* [152, p. 187]. He cited not only popes but also pop singers, but all the songs Farmer sang were of pragmatic solidarity. Physicians could accompany patients to health and justice. Physicians could partner with communities and families. He made the hospital sound like a kind of sanctified union hall where the indigent and the wealthy, the ill and the well, worked together.

Farmer also pointed back to other physicians in the same lineage. One of his own heroes was Rudolf Virchow, the nineteenth-century anthropologist and physician who founded social medicine. Virchow was a pathologist who developed the modern autopsy, founded the fields of cellular and comparative pathology, and discovered (and named) the processes that governed clotting. Virchow was such a gifted scientist that four parts of the human body—Virchow's angle, line, node, and spaces—bear his name. But despite his understanding of disease, he insisted that the leading cause of medical illness was social inequality. Virchow knew the body and the community. Sometimes, Virchow believed, the best medical treatment was a political action. Virchow, Farmer liked to say, called physicians "the natural attorneys of the poor," the people who directly encounter the poor in their vulnerability and can best advocate for their social needs [153, p. 234].

. . .

Catherine Ard, the fourth-year student, is trying to make natural attorneys. All year, the LIC students worked on the service learning projects established by Catherine. Toward the end of the year, she returns to a Thursday chalice exercise with mixed news. Students loved the curriculum. The experience at the youth homeless shelter worked out. However, the Somali Bantu refugee partnership fell apart. Catherine could not say entirely why. Coordinating schedules, building relationships, and navigating cultures are more difficult than building a lecture, but that did not fully explain it. She wondered if she had found the right community partners. She wondered what it meant for a community partner to be the right one. She asked how you make sure a community benefits from a student's learning.

When Catherine speaks, she echoes Farmer's invocation of Virchow. It sounds like a different path for future physicians than the one Flexner charted, forming med students into natural attorneys who encounter the vulnerable poor and become their advocates and companions. Is it possible? Or should you recruit med students, like Ford, from marginalized communities themselves? Do you train physicians to be scientific professionals like Flexner or natural attorneys like Virchow? Med students who had not just visited the homes of patients but grown up alongside them might be better able to serve communities like the Somali Bantu refugees.

. . .

Mackenzie was one of the students most eager to address social determinants as a natural attorney. Before she enrolled in medical school, she considered a doctorate in public health. Public health focused on preventing disease before it started, increasing access to care, and addressing the social determinants of health. Although she settled on medical school, Mackenzie was determined to undertake public health training along the way.

In her first few years of med school, she published a blog for med school aspirants, and it was full of observations (*most of the lecturing faculty are specialists who try to recruit you for their field*) and encouragement (*don't forget that you are good enough*). But the theme she sounded most often was injustice.

As it stands, the culture of medicine is largely entangled with the culture of money and capitalism in medicine.

My general philosophy is that I should listen before I speak so that I can fully understand a situation, especially when it comes to advocacy.

I strongly believe that our societal problems largely occur because our culture values some lives more than others.

We can't all find the cure for cancer or stop a war or fix the system, but we can all speak up when we see small injustices happening in our own spheres of influence.

To stand up, to listen, to value everyone, to speak up—these were the actions a medical student needed to take.

Mackenzie knew that you could measure equity when assessing health and that most measures reveal shocking levels of inequity; the differential experiences of Black patients and physicians were the issues that troubled her most.

The students frequently repeated a public health maxim—*When white people get a cold, Black people get pneumonia*—that emphasizes how the same biological processes affect communities differentially. Race, while no biological difference, is a profound predictor of health. They could rattle off the comparisons. Black people are twice as likely to die in pregnancy. Black infants are three times more likely to die. Black children are twice as likely to develop asthma. Black adults develop chronic diseases—cancer, hypertension, kidney disease, obesity—sooner than white adults and die younger. Black people are also more likely to experience the social determinants—poverty, homelessness, unemployment, incarceration, food insecurity, discrimination—that undermine and erode health. When they seek care, they are more likely to be uninsured or publicly insured than white Americans, and their care is distorted and limited by algorithms built into the EHR that send patients down different care pathways because of their race [154, 155]. In the face of these differences, researchers conceptualize racism itself as a cause of health disparities [156].

As she neared the end of her LIC year, Mackenzie decided it was time to learn more about how to improve the health of a community by earning an MPH. "I went back and forth between doing it now versus later as part of a fellowship or as an attending someday. And then, I just thought, 'If I don't do it now, it's never going to happen.'" She decided to extend the duration of medical school so she could earn an MPH after her LIC year, return for her final year of med school, and then seek her Match with an internal medicine residency that would train her clinically to address the social determinants of health.

. . .

Ford was born a natural attorney, staying on the Virchow path her whole life, even as institutional medicine tried to knock her off. At the end of her career, she recalled that when she initially applied for her medical license, she was told that she had two strikes against her: "First off you're a lady. Second, you're colored." Her response: "I fought like a tiger against those things" [151].

By 1950, Ford's eyesight was failing her, but her fight was paying off. She built a practice. She learned to speak eight languages so that she could understand and be understood by her patients. She was widely appreciated by the region's poor and working class. She, after all, delivered seven thousand of their children—two generations.

They loved her for caring for them in their homes, especially staying for hours with a laboring mother. Decades later, a former patient still remembered Dr. Ford. "She had the softest, silkiest hands of anyone I'd ever known. . . . I can close my eyes and still see her coming into the house. Her chauffeur would wait for hours. Dr. Ford would stay overnight. She would clean everything and stay until the birth. I remember her face" [157, p. 92].

Patients remembered her face because she was present in their home when no other physician would cross the threshold. They remember her sleeping on the couch when a baby refused to come. They remember her using delicate hands instead of unforgiving forceps to coax a baby. They remember that when she raised the shades, neighbors knew that Dr. Ford had delivered another child. They remember that on the way home she would often stop at the neighborhood grocer, where she had a standing order: if she raised one finger, the grocer would deliver the family a single bag; two fingers meant two bags of groceries for Ford's newest patient and their family. They remember that Ford understood and acted on the social determinants of health long ago.

Ford made her home among Denver's immigrant communities, practicing as a natural attorney until two weeks before her death from kidney failure on October 14, 1952.

The state's medical institutions made a home for her only begrudgingly. The only hospital that ever appointed her to their faculty was Denver Health, and it did so only a quarter century into her career. She spent her career as a solo practitioner working parallel to the discriminatory systems of institutional medicine. Her place in the state was even more singular. A full half century after she began practicing, she was one of only seven Black physicians and still the state's only Black female physician [11, 151, 157].

In that century, as well as this one, when Black people sought care, they were less likely to receive care from a person who could help them flourish. This was another consequence of the *Flexner Report*. Flexner believed that Black physicians should be educated—he admired how the medical schools at Howard and Meharry did so—but he made no calls for the integration of white medical schools. In the report's 346 pages, Flexner allotted only a page and a half to discussing the education of Black medical students. Its seven paragraphs mention the risks posed by infectious disease to Black people, but never the risks posed by Jim Crow, or the risks of separate but (supposedly) equal schooling, or the risks of measuring the dreams of Black med students by his definition of merit [158, 159]. Instead, he advised steering most Black students toward careers in public health rather than medicine. "A well taught negro sanitarian will be immensely useful; an essentially untrained negro wearing an M.D. degree is dangerous. Make-believe in the matter of negro medical schools is therefore intolerable. Even good intention helps but little to change their aspect. The negro needs good schools rather than many schools, schools to which the more promising of the race can be sent to receive a substantial education in which hygiene rather than surgery, for example, is strongly accentuated" [14, p. 180]. Flexner circumscribed the roles of Black students— sanitarians instead of surgeons—while harshly concluding that most medical schools for Black students were in "no position to make any contribution of value" and should be shuttered [14, p. 180]. And so they were, ensuring that medical education for Black physicians would be separate and unequal for the rest of the twentieth century.

The Flexner-era reforms that spoke so fleetingly of "the general interest of a community" turned a segregated nineteenth-century profession into a shuttered twentieth-century profession [158]. By the middle of the twentieth century, 80 percent of Black American physicians were graduating from the only two schools for Black medical students, Howard and Meharry, that survived Flexner. The other one-hundred-plus medical schools, following the *Flexner Report*'s injunction to reform without integration, produced the scant remaining 20 percent [160, 161].

By the time the LIC students were in med school, 8.4 percent of medical school applicants, 7.1 percent of medical school acceptees, 6.2 percent of medical school graduates, 5.0 percent of all practicing physicians, and 3.6 percent of full-time medical school faculty identified as Black or African American [162]. At every step in a physician's journey, the number of Black physicians decreased. At a place like Denver Health, where only four physicians identified as Black or African American, it left the medical staff without the best natural attorneys for many of its patients.

As much as the students want to follow in the footsteps of pioneers like Ford, they also see that they are still taking half steps. The LIC surely takes a half step beyond the standard biomedical education model codified by Flexner, the textbook of the body. The LIC helps the students take a version of the half step taken by Sabin, who learned the textbook of the body and then learned how to improve the health of the community through public health, but in the beginning of their career. The LIC surely accelerates the timeline followed by Sabin, but the textbook of the community is not a truly collaborative model of care. Any textbook still implies a learn-and-apply model, rather than a collaborative creation with a community. The students can stand up against injustice, participate in service learning, follow patients over time, and earn public health degrees, but they are assigned to visit the homes of patients, instead of living alongside them.

. . .

Thurline was the first patient Mackenzie met in her home. Thurline had cirrhosis, a scarring of the liver after repeated injuries, so she needed frequent medical care, the kind of condition that is promising for a medical student seeking to follow a patient during the LIC year. Mackenzie followed Thurline all the way to her home, where she received the kind of hello that doctors rarely get, the patient's welcome rather than the professional's greeting.

"It was really impressive to me that despite all of her health issues and the challenges of her past, she was just kind and wonderful, so I followed her closely. I did a home visit with her and got to know her and her friend who always drove her places.

"She didn't have a bed because a month earlier she had fallen and hit her head and got blood all over her bed. So they got rid of it. She'd just been sleeping in her recliner and then on the floor for a month. She had a really low level of mobility."

Where you sleep is the kind of detail that obviously shapes your health, but doctors rarely ask about. Doctors typically project what they know of home onto the homes of their patients. Doctors unconsciously imagine arrangements—furniture, finances, family—that resemble what they know. When a medical student makes a home visit, she replaces those projections with reality.

"At her house, she had a list of all the things she needed to do for her health. She had this big issue with potassium, going back and forth with her medications. She had this list from one of her doctors about potassium up on her wall. She'd very religiously keep up with things like potassium and her lactulose dosing and all the things doctors asked her to do. She was working really hard." Mackenzie admired how Thurline followed doctors' orders but was still worried about her health.

Thurline bit and picked at her nails so aggressively that they were torn and bleeding, as she fretted over what she had lost and was still losing. "She would always wear gloves around her grandkids, so that they wouldn't know or see. She wanted to make sure they had what they needed." And her grandkids weren't the only ones she cared for. "She would ask about how I was doing and how her other doctors were doing. She cared about us."

Mackenzie was able to see how Thurline endured loss by thinking about other people, as well as how hard a person must work at being a patient, only when she visited Thurline's home.

. . .

Home visits are a start, but students like Catherine and Mackenzie and teachers like Adams have concluded that medicine must change who is in the room. Adams wants medical students who speak languages other than English and understand cultures beyond the meritocracy. In the meantime, Adams assigns the students she does have to serve patients of different cultures. She endorses curricular pilots like Catherine's service-learning curriculum. She sends students like Mackenzie to visit patients in their homes. She trains students who aspire to be natural attorneys for the people most in need.

But Adams knows that medicine needs more natural attorneys who, like Dr. Ford, truly belong to the communities in which they practice.

Toward the end of her life, Dr. Ford wrote a letter, again pleading for membership in the Colorado Medical Society: "I do general practice work among all classes + races—many are in the low income group." On January 3, 1950, she was finally allowed to join the Colorado Medical Society, which led to membership in the American Medical Association [163, pp. 34–35]. But it came too late to alter her career. She never became a faculty member at the state's medical school, which graduated its first Black women—Deborah Green and LaRae H. Washington—in 1975, over a century after Ford's birth [164, p. 632]. Medicine is still missing many of the natural attorneys capable of really following in Dr. Ford's footsteps toward a truly collaborative model of medicine.

Chapter 24

GRATITUDE EXERCISES

*M*EGAN KALATA WAS WARNED about the Match. "You get a lot of very intelligent, but maybe not always emotionally intelligent, people and you put them all in a room together with very high emotions. And then, you don't provide enough tissues, and everybody's crying. And you don't know if it's happy tears or sad tears, and it's just very strange."

Parents usually fly in to watch the tears fall. But this year, parental flights are storm grounded. A bomb cyclone, the most powerful storm in Colorado's recorded history—a pressure drop of 970 millibars that is the winter equivalent of a Category 2 hurricane—is sweeping in snow and sweeping away the students' plans. The next day's festivities are already canceled.

Tomorrow is Match Day for the class ahead of the current LIC students, the day friends like Catherine Ard learn which residency they secured. Catherine and her classmates spent an entire year applying to dozens of programs, flying about the country to the programs that granted the interviews, agonizing over how to rank the programs, and then waiting, waiting, waiting for the third Friday of March. After all that travel, Catherine wants nothing more than to stay put. She has unfinished business with her patients, her preceptors, and her community. She loves the local general internal medicine program for allowing her to maintain continuity with them all. She hopes her Match reads "home."

Whatever it says, Catherine will receive her Match at the same time as every other physician aspirant in the country: 1:00 p.m. eastern standard time. The Match determines the specialty they will practice, impacts the career they will have, and influences the place they will live, as more than half of all resident physicians will practice in the state in which they completed residency [165].

Each school serves up its Match differently. At some schools, the dress code is costume party. At other schools, it is business casual. At Colorado, it is formal, fitting for the downtown ballroom setting. Partners and friends come to lend support as the students stare at an envelope for fifteen minutes while a dean talks. When finally permitted, students tear open their envelopes simultaneously, speed-read their fates, and run even faster about the room to share their Match with their peers, or exit as quickly as possible to shield their disappointment.

Even though this year's formal event is canceled, the Match goes on. Megan believes in celebrating, so she planned an informal party for four friends. She will bake and decorate a homemade cake.

Maggie Kriz, imagining her own Match Day, says, "No matter what happens when I open that envelope, I am going to cry."

As the students daydream about their future Matches, Dr. Adams, looking at the clock, proposes that, since the next lecturer is herself delayed by the storm, they move up their last team-based learning exercise of the year.

"Do you want to use the chalice, or should we break into teams using a different method? Who played in the snow yesterday?"

No one raises a hand.

"Which of you wore pajamas all day yesterday?"

Maggie's and Mallory's hands go up. Not enough for a team.

Megan proposes, "We should make teams by favorite organ."

Adams asks, "Who's favorite organ is the liver? Whose favorite organ is the heart?"

Too many students favor the liver over the heart—it regenerates itself and metabolizes everything, while the heart wins all the metaphorical glory but is, to a med student, a muscular pump—to form equal teams.

Itzam Marin proposes, "We can do it by antibiotics. Who will prescribe a seven-day course? Who a ten-day course?"

"Okay," Adams tries, "Which of you would prescribe a ten-day course for cellulitis?"

No one's hands stir.

"I've trained you all too well! Okay, who made hot chocolate yesterday?"

Only Itzam raises his hand.

Adams tries again: "What about your favorite season: summer or winter?"

There's a lot of chatter; no teams form.

"How do you like to spend snow days?"

Now she has a dividing line, the formation of three teams, based on how they prefer to spend the unexpected benefit of a snow day. Partnered off, the students enter easily into the assignment's rhythm: pretest of their knowledge; score the pretest; explain the missed questions; case-based exercise with partners.

Today's case is a forty-nine-year-old HIV+ man with chest pain, cough, subjective fever, and chills. The teams review the history and EKG for fifteen minutes. Tachycardia and tachypnea. EKG with diffuse ST elevations. Adams asks each team first for the top three most likely diagnoses and then for the information that supports each diagnosis. She spools out a little more information and asks the students to expand the possible diagnoses. Working together, all the students settle on endocarditis, pneumothorax, gastroesophageal reflux disease, esophagitis, pancreatitis, aortic dissection, pneumonia, and asthma. It's an exhausting—but not exhaustive—list of ailments.

"What would you like to do in the first ten minutes while this patient is before you?"

The students suggest labs and a chest X-ray. Adams expected that, so she nods, pulls up the chest X-ray, and asks the students to read its inverted portrait of the shadows of the body and reconsider their differential diagnoses. A student volunteers a reading.

"I see a little bit of tracheal deviation to the right. . . . Not being able to appreciate the costophrenic silhouette. . . . Our diagnosis was pericardial tamponade. We wanted to do a bedside echo with a pericardiocentesis needle."

Adams ask, "What if the echo tech is backed up?

The student offers, "Point of care ultrasound?"

"You don't have that. You have the exam. What exam finding is characteristic?"

The student fumbles. Adams gives the official name, pulsus paradoxus, and then plays a video describing how the heart's second Korsakoff sound does, in a healthy individual, and does not, in a person with pulsus, disappear with inspiration. Normal: *lub-dub*. Pulsus: *lub-lub*. Adams returns the students back to their teams, so the students can bounce diagnostic possibilities off each other.

Ten minutes later, Adams calls them back to the board to discuss next steps for the workup of the patient's pericarditis. Pericarditis is a state—inflammation of the fibrous sac that encases the heart—so first they create a differential for the reasons it could be inflamed: idiopathic, viral, rheumatologic, bacterial, fungal, malignant, and more.

The students return to their groups with a new EKG to interpret. None of them can puzzle it out. Adams has made her point. The students have more to learn. Being a physician means there is always more to learn.

"I wanted to share this case with you because I learned so much from it. The patient had stage III pericarditis." Adams explains that it induced peculiar, transient EKG findings that she understood only with the assistance of a cardiologist.

"Sometimes the EKGs normalize, then you get abnormal EKGs when the symptoms resolve. It's a really interesting course. You treat it with colchicine until it resolves."

The students return to the case to seek the underlying diagnosis. They eventually land on syphilis, the disease so famous for the multiple ways it can present clinically that generations of medical educators called it the Great Impostor and featured it in clinical reasoning exercises because it encouraged consideration of so many kinds of pathology. Osler, the physician so esteemed by Flexner, wrote, "I often tell my students that it is the only disease which they require to study thoroughly. Know syphilis in all its manifestations and relations, and all other things clinical will be added unto you" [36, p. 140]. Adams added it unto her own students, so she can conclude the case and the year with a doctor's farewell that drops a hint about a change awaiting her too.

"I am in the process of saying goodbye to all my HIV patients and I met with him last week and he asked me, 'But aren't I the one in your textbook?' I had to explain to him that it was just a team-based learning case, but now you will remember him."

Adams is terminating with her patients in the HIV clinic as she takes on more work at the medical school. Her teamwork earned her a new job. It is how teams work in medicine. If your team proves you can do the work, you get more work, and then you must leave behind some of the people with whom you have worked. It's true for the students as well. They must break up with each other—and, like Adams, with their patients—so they can take on their next work.

. . .

Before Adams and Mallory see a clinic patient, Adams reminds Mallory that this will be her last time to see the patient. Mallory always knew she would terminate, but she suddenly felt unprepared. The relationship meant a great deal to her, but it had boundaries. Today, she will enforce the final one.

"I didn't know quite what to say. I started by saying, 'This may be the last time I see you.' I wasn't sure how she was going to react, because perhaps our relationship has been more meaningful for me than it has been for her. She asked me where I was going, and I explained that I would be applying for residency. She wished me good luck and thanked me for being involved in her care. It felt silly to hear her thanking me—really I should be thanking her for letting me be involved with her care! I did tell her this, and that I truly learned so much from her this past year. What I didn't tell her—and maybe I should have—is that she is the patient who ultimately convinced me to go into Internal Medicine. She helped me realize that I would hate to go my entire life without having longitudinal relationships with patients like her."

Mallory had seen the patient from an initial presentation through a diagnosis and on to treatment. During this journey, her role shifted: sometimes a learner, sometimes a companion, soon a physician.

"I was there on her hardest days in the hospital when she expressed fears of getting a pacemaker, and then I was there on the other side of that pacemaker when her symptoms had nearly disappeared."

In their time together, they grew fond of each other.

"We spent hours in the hospital learning about each other's lives—talking about our families, our aspirations, and our fears. Each time I saw her in clinic, she'd ask me how my last shelf exam went and I'd ask her about her daughters. She really allowed me to see her as more than just a patient, and she in turn saw me as more than just a medical student. She is a patient that I will carry with me for the rest of my life."

And that life would be different. Some experiences change what we know and who we are. When a medical student selects her specialty, she selects her transformative experience. An internist knows different things than an anesthesiologist and behaves differently. They overlap in their love for numbers. If every sentence you speak has a data point in it, anesthesiology and internal medicine will both be comforting. Mallory had initially thought she would be doing anesthesiology, but it was too focused on the textbook of the body. She is choosing internal medicine because of her experience with this patient and others. And yet she makes her goodbyes so she can say her hellos to her future patients. She does it by saying thank you.

Giving thanks regularly makes a habit of gratitude; Maggie has it mastered.

A few hours before graduation, she is like a thank-you machine. Every story she tells reflects her gratitude to someone or another—even when the story is hard.

She shares a piece she wrote about one of those hard stories. It was her last OB-GYN clinic. She was kind of relieved; OB-GYN was not her passion. "I think when you experienced that, it's sort of scary when you're like, 'Whoa, I thought I had an idea of what I wanted to do and now I realize that that's not at all what I want to do.'" She began the year thinking that her future was as an obstetrician, but midway through the year she realized that she was not excited on her OB-GYN clinic days.

"I think that if I wanted to go into obstetrics, it would have been a better path to go in the midwifery side of things. I think that vaginal childbirth is amazing and it was incredible to deliver babies. It was also really messy. There were things I saw that left me saying, 'Oh God, like, now I'm scared to have children.' Especially when you do deliveries of women who have gestational diabetes and their baby is 10 pounds. I just don't like the model. I don't like C-sections. It feels very barbaric to like rip into a woman's uterus, really legitimately ripping into her uterus."

Maggie ended the year on the other side of her obstetrics dream, but she was very pleased to see her last patient of the day. She had followed the patient all year. The woman had experienced multiple miscarriages but was pregnant again, visiting for a routine pregnancy examination.

"It was an OB visit, just like any other—we began by asking about vaginal bleeding, loss of fluid, contractions, nausea, but then my patient said: 'I don't feel pregnant.'"

Maggie reassured her that every pregnancy is unique but said they would listen to make sure everything was okay.

"I put the Doppler on her belly, pointed it towards her pelvis, and for the first time in my schooling, found nothing."

Again, she reassured the patient that it can be difficult to hear a heartbeat at this stage, so they could try an ultrasound.

"Now, our worst fears were realized: we could not see the beautiful and complex yet simple flutter inside the baby's chest. We told the mother that the baby was lost, that she had miscarried for the fourth time."

Maggie thought of other experiences she'd had with babies who had died before birth. She had knitted hats for some of them. She had mourned some of them.

"It is impossible, when you share such a profound and human connection, to not be overcome with empathy. But having lived this experience allowed me to connect with this mother, to empathize in a unique way only those who have experienced such tragedy can understand. I stayed with her for over an hour, giving her what she needed—at times silence, at times a shoulder to cry on."

She left the clinic ruminating on the pain this woman was feeling. She remembered a passage from one of her favorite novels in which a father consoles his son. "Nature has cunning ways of finding our weakest spot. Just remember: I am here. Right now you may not want to feel anything, maybe you never wanted to feel anything. . . . In your place, if there is pain, nurse it, and if there is a flame, don't snuff it out, don't be brutal with it" [166, p. 224]. Maggie had been wounded by medical training. She stayed with it, let it change her, let it alter her dream. She felt all the feels. Now she feels thanks.

"What I hope to take away from the hundreds of hours with my preceptors and patients is that we are all human beings and we must remember to treat each other with compassion, honor, and dignity." Maggie knew who she wanted to be as a physician: "to approach each patient with an open heart and a focused mind, to be the person who will stay with a patient even when it is difficult, to be a trusted confidant and a knowledgeable provider, but fundamentally and most importantly to connect with patients on a human level and to remember that more things bind us than separate us."

Maggie is navigating being a person and a physician at the same time, through all the fluids, through all the pains. When asked how, she laughs and says, "I'm still figuring that out."

. . .

The shared goodbyes and hellos at the end of the LIC year occur a week later. The sun has melted the snow, warmed the air, and allowed a different set of parents into town. Graduation from the LIC is an evening affair in a break room on the fifth floor of the hospital's administration building, a building not nearly as august as the ballroom where they are scheduled to receive their own Match a year later. But this break room has a full-sized kitchen.

This is good, because there is even more food than usual and more people around the table. LIC preceptors, students, and their families are chatting between bites; food is the universal material expression of gratitude.

Itzam excitedly introduces his wife. Andrea has red hair, an open face, and a gravid abdomen. After he got sick, he says things changed.

They couldn't wait. Now, they're expecting. Andrea politely shakes hands, a little surprised by the introduction. A very med student hello, introducing someone with their health status. Itzam will take less strenuous courses around her September due date, then bear down for several advanced courses to secure a surgical residency. He stayed true to ophthalmology, the right blend of clinic and operating room, continuity and acute, body and community. They have family in Texas and Mexico, none in Colorado. He dreams of someday helping patients in his native country, and Texas is closer. He says, "We love Colorado but are interested in seeing more of the country," code for *I might leave.*

The faculty will stay. The clinical preceptors and the Thursday teachers are all here. They compare notes from their own training days, realizing where paths crossed at academic medical centers near and far. At the beginning of the year, the faculty were the only people in the classroom sessions who knew the answers. Now at the end of the year, the faculty and students are learning together. Over the course of the year, the students' knowledge and problem-solving have grown enough that they are teaching specialists about the parts of general medicine the faculty had forgotten or never learned. They have become almost-doctors. They are the future of medicine.

An hour into the evening, Dr. Adams stands before the assembled group, asks everyone to find their seats, and, just when the students think she will introduce yet another case for them to solve, starts her thank-yous. The student's families, the faculty, and, of course, Oatis. Kris and Jen, Jen and Kris, the duo that stays together as each cohort of students change. Then Adams raises her hand to the ceiling before diving it low into the silvered bowl, saying, "I will use the chalice of opportunity to award the certificates."

She fishes out Megan's name, and Megan comes up to the front of the room. Adams calls up Megan's preceptors too; every physician who stands for her is a woman. At the beginning of the year, Megan wondered if she had a future in medicine. Now, she is standing in its midst, choosing between two possible futures as a physician who cares for women, family medicine or obstetrics. Adams tells the audience about the speculum valentine. Megan smiles and shrugs. "I love crafts."

Then she keeps quiet as the faculty speak of her. Dr. Lowdermilk from psychiatry praises how she knows what to ask and what not to ask. Dr. Jaiswal—the carrier of coffee—from surgery praises her for being able to consent a patient better than any student she had ever worked with. "I am so pleased you can do a perfect breast exam and know that will be such a good thing for the women you see." Her family medicine preceptor says, "Even in our first week together, she jumped right in. She went in on her own, on nights and weekends, to be with our patients. The patients really appreciated that. You have this amazing aura of confidence and compassion." Dr. Cleeves—the creator of the needlepoint—from internal medicine is the last to speak but the first to cry. "I've already cried in front of her this week. I've worked with her lots of places this year"; she daubs her face and continues, "What is going to stick with me is your warmth." Megan smiles widely as she silently dispenses hugs. Her mother and sister flash the same smiles from the audience.

Sarah Bardwell steps up next; she is eventually bound to family medicine but will take a gap year first. She is increasingly certain that she is uncertain. She cannot follow a straight path through medical training. Adams starts, "Sarah was sick with the flu. Now her preceptors are too, so we have some written comments from them." After the laughter and the groans die down, Adams praises Sarah's commitment and grit. "You have an incredible ability to connect with patients and an incredible compassion for the human experience. When I think of you, you embody the word 'altruism,' and I will remember you that way." Her family medicine preceptor praises Sarah for her "fierce commitment to being a humanistic physician even when the system almost forces us to do otherwise. She reminded me to be a better physician for my patients, even when I am facing similar pressures." Kulasekaran reads comments praising her empathy and interviewing skills and how she thinks about patients all the time.

Adams calls up Maggie and announces that she is headed to medicine-pediatrics. Dr. Frank, her preceptor and the assistant program director for the medicine-pediatrics residency, cheers. (All evening, the faculty cheer when a student's future is announced as their own specialty and boo when they hear that a beloved student is headed elsewhere.) With tears in her eyes, Maggie stands next to Adams, who praises her energy, her enthusiasm, and her ability to knit remarkable things during class. "I loved watching her make amazing things and develop this incredible love of children and adolescents." Frank, excited to recruit her first LIC student into med-peds, enthuses, "She is the most motivated student I have worked with. She wants to figure everything out for herself. She lights up when she sees a teenager, the more complicated the better. Patients truly trust her." Dr. Stichman steps forward and gives Maggie a card, a knitting pattern, and a shawl she knitted herself. Maggie drapes the thank-you shawl around her shoulders, and it is quickly a little damp with tears. Stichman says, "Whenever I travel anywhere, I get yarn, and it always has a story. When you get yarn somewhere, make something somewhere, it has a story. This is the yarn I got during my fourth year of med school. I hope it has stories for you." As Stichman hands over the ball of yarn, Maggie's fiancé, Sean, grins from the audience.

Itzam steps forward, and Adams observes, "He is going into a career in ophthalmology. Even though he knew that pretty early on, he really cared where patients came from, who anchored them, and what had meaning for them. I know he will carry that forward. When I think about the goal of this program, that is as important as anything, as well as your deep commitment to our marginalized patients." She praises his ability to do so, even through a thyroid storm. Lowdermilk testifies: "You found what made the patients proud, and that was really special. Often, in medicine we tell people what they are doing wrong, and you told them what they were doing right." Lowdermilk does, however, report that Itzam disappointed one of her patients by being unavailable to marry her granddaughter. While Itzam blushes, an internist says he was especially helpful with their Spanish-speaking patients. Itzam would enter a room and spend an hour explaining the situation. When she entered, the internist says patients would pull her aside to whisper, "This guy is really good. He could be my doctor."

Mallory steps forward. A pediatrician introduces her as "a quiet, gentle force, the kind of student who makes you a better teacher and you do not even realize it. And I thank you for it. She is better at applying feedback than any student I have ever worked with. That will serve you well throughout your life and career. We work with a large immigrant population, and they told you things that they would not disclose to anyone else, even though they had been coming to our clinic for years." Lowdermilk keeps it simple. "I am not sure how clinic will run without you. I usually keep a list of questions that a student missed, questions that I have to ask after the student finishes. You kept me quiet in the room because you asked everything that needed to be asked." Now Adams finishes. "Each year, I only get to work with one of the students in my internal medicine clinic. This year, it was you. You give truly exceptional patient care. You have an incredible bedside manner. You are so patient with even our most challenging patients. I just trust you completely."

As Mackenzie Garcia steps up last, Adams calls out her "incredible dedication to the underserved and her patients. She has this incredible energy for learning. I will miss you a lot, especially at 6:30, when I am leaving, and you are still talking to your patients. You will be a beacon of humanism." An emergency medicine physician says, "Our patients, and we see all kinds, loved her. We work as a team in the emergency department and we do well when we work as a team. And I saw incredible growth from you this year. I remember your first presentation and your last presentation." The emergency medicine physician rues that Mackenzie is headed to internal medicine after her public health training. Not so Dr. Sacro, an internist who could not attend but sent a note praising Mackenzie for always finding what is interesting about every patient and gifted her a few lines from Rupi Kaur:

> we all move forward when
> we recognize how resilient
> and striking the women
> around us are. [167, p. 191]

After the students, family, and faculty finish their cheering, they eat green cake meant for a different kind of feast. At her request, Adams's husband collected a cake for the event, and their nine-year-old twin boys thought the best one was a Saint Patrick's Day cake from the grocery store's discounted pastry section. No matter. As people grow more familiar while eating week-old cake that stains their teeth green, you see gratitude, the kind of warm appreciation that turns a hospital break room into a place where true encounters occur. Gratitude gathered around the students tonight, taking the form of an exquisite courtesy toward each other, of valentine's cards, of draped shawls, of poetry, of discounted green cake. The students were honored but said very little. There were no humblebrag acceptance speeches, no valedictory pronouncements. Graduation was an extended gratitude exercise.

Psychiatrists prescribe those sometimes.

Rx: Write down five things for which you are grateful. Repeat once weekly.

Psychiatrists tell patients that writing about what you are thankful for—instead of what has merely occurred or, worse, what bothers you—will reduce anxiety, depression, and pain while increasing energy, sleep, and well-being. Adams warned students to defend against the three *D*'s that threaten a physician. When the students savor the good in the present and imagine good futures, they move from defense to offense. They flourish.

Chapter 25

RANK LISTS

$\mathcal{M}$EGAN KALATA MAPPED OUT several different decisions before finalizing her rank list for the Match. Since it's now up to the algorithm to realize her dreams, she and her friends are texting each other their anxious nightmares. Will their envelopes bear bad news, be blank, or deliver something bizarre?

"The other night I had a dream that in order to Match, I had to prove myself by having a home birth. But I told them I wasn't pregnant, and so I didn't know how I was going to do that. And they said I just had to figure it out. I was stressed I wasn't going to Match because I wasn't going to be able to pass the test."

To birth herself—this is the type of dream a med student has.

Her waking dream for the Match is more realistic but just as anxious. She applied in both family medicine and OB-GYN, so she is worried about where she will train and what kind of doctor it will make her. "My rank list ended up having both OB and family in that top five or six, so there are places in both specialties that I would be happy. Either way, I'll be very happy for some reasons and there will also be a part of me that will be sad about the pieces I'm leaving behind from whichever specialty I don't end up in."

Since Megan's Match will embrace one specialty and foreclose the other, she looks for residency programs that bridge her interests. She wants OB programs that care for the underserved and teach health advocacy and policy. She wants family medicine programs with more female patients in which she can perform more obstetrical procedures. She wants her right balance between body and community.

Megan must decide, without knowing precisely who she will become after her decision. Some decisions are like that, changing what we know and who we are. When a medical student selects her specialty, she is selecting an experience that will transform her. An obstetrician-gynecologist knows different things than a family practitioner and behaves differently in the hospital. If Megan matches in OB-GYN, it will mean no more well-child checks, no more school physicals, no more seeing male patients. A med student cannot know what it will be like to give that up, or to take on the activities only an obstetrician-gynecologist takes on. Colpos, cone biopsies, Leep procedures, and so many pap smears. It is all knowledge. And it will all change a student. And the student cannot know how it will change them until they undertake the training.

The philosopher L. A. Paul calls these kinds of activities transformative experiences, big choices that will result in changes we cannot fully predict. Paul gives examples: receiving a cochlear implant after being born deaf, getting married, having a first child, and becoming a vampire. "With one swift, painless bite, you'll be permanently transformed into an elegant and fabulous creature of the night. As a member of the undead, your life will be completely different." Those kinds of experiences, Paul observes, are intense, overwhelming, and life-changing in ways you can never fully predict. Paul names only one profession as a similar kind of life-changing experience. "Becoming a doctor requires a high level of commitment, focus and planning, not to mention luck and hard work. . . . Medical school and residency are grueling experiences that require you to set aside other pursuits and focus almost entirely on your training and performance" [168, pp. 98–99].

Only doctoring, in her account, is like becoming a parent or a vampire. Parents, vampires, and physicians—all are transformed in the middle of the night. It is at night that they soothe some of the crying, bleed others dry, and mend the ones they can.

When a medical student selects her specialty, she is choosing whether she wants to discover a new way of living, say, life as an ob-gyn or life as a family practitioner. Megan is choosing to become the kind of person—without knowing what that will be like—that her experiences will make her into. To help her decide, she talks to friends, peers, and especially LIC alumni, because she knows they share her interests. They prepared her for interviews and suggested programs to which she could apply.

Between the two specialties, she applied to ninety residencies, entering the market in pursuit of many possible Matches. Interview requests trickled in over her email, and she usually had only minutes, at most hours, to respond before the interview spots were claimed by other applicants.

"When interviews started coming out, I was doing an away GYN rotation. I was worried about that classic thing that you hear people being in the OR and getting offered an interview and then getting out and not having time to respond to it. Luckily, my sister said, 'I can watch your email for you.' We had a Google Sheet with days marked in red if I really didn't want to be traveling somewhere or interviewing somewhere because there was something going on in Denver or days marked in yellow if I thought I'd be in the Midwest."

Megan limited travel costs where she could, staying with family and alumni, but still spent around $3,000 to apply and another $3,000 to interview at twenty-nine programs.

Now, she awaits her own fate. The official Match is on a Friday, but on Monday morning applicants find out if they matched anywhere at all. That morning, every applicant receives an email declaring either that the algorithm has assigned them to a program or that they are unmatched.

Megan plans to be at home, in full professional dress, in case she falls among the unmatched. If she receives the dreaded "We're sorry, but you did not match to any position" message, she will have no residency position awaiting her on the other side of all her labors. The prefix suggests how a student's work can be undone, leaving them unapproved, unsubstantiated, an un-physician. But there is a narrow path to escape the negative fate of the un-. An unmatched student can embark on a four-day frantic effort to secure a spot with a program that is similarly unmatched. It's a maddening game of musical chairs for a doctor's future, a disheartening trick, in which applicants send CVs to programs they never visited, while feelings of regret and failure roil inside them [169]. If no program reaches out, an unmatched student can apply for an additional year of medical school to mask their failure or graduate into a gap year and apply again. But a gap year often widens into a career-ending chasm—less than one half of the unmatched will match in subsequent years—leaving a doctor who is never known as a physician, unable to practice or care for the sick, opening a gap between their training and their identity [170]. To avoid the gap, an applicant refreshes her email obsessively, calls in every favor she can recall, and pleads with every deity she can countenance. If an unmatched program reaches out, a student's shame gives way to a furious Google-stalk to understand the program, an internal debate about how willing they are to move somewhere remote to be near their dream, and then a quick conversation where both sides are deciding if they want to spend at least a year together. While some of the programs offer full residencies of three years or more, most of the slots are for one-year standalone internships, the resident physician's equivalent of entering the temp economy. The whole awkward game used to go by a descriptive name, the Scramble, which reflected the frantic pace befitting a medical education maneuver that determined—in mere hours—what kind of doctor they would become and where, after discovering that their first choice and all the choices after that had not selected them. Recently, the name has been softened to the acronymic SOAP, the Match's Supplemental Offer and Acceptance Program, but every applicant and program is desperate to avoid its version of cleaning up.

She will wait for an email with the subject line "Did I Match?," click it open, speed-read its contents, and activate one of two plans. If matched, she will text Dr. Adams. If unmatched, she will text Dr. Adams, drive to the university, and begin the frantic search of the unmatched applicant for a spot in an unfilled program.

Megan has done what she can to secure a Match. Now, she can only wait for Monday and plan for Friday. If Monday goes well, her twin sister and her parents will attend the Match. Her boyfriend will not be able to attend. He is, himself, a family medicine intern and will be working. Depending on what the Match decides, they could wind up in the same program, be together long-distance, or break up. Their future will be determined by the market.

. . .

The fourth year of med school is advertised as the easiest school year since kindergarten. Everything that you learn will be relearned the following year in greater detail, so don't sweat the details. The point is to become socialized in preparation for your real training, so don't forget that the playground is as important as the classroom. But the advertising misleads. Children learn more in kindergarten than adults care to remember, and its socialization is an oft-painful process with sudden shifts between moments of inclusion and exclusion.

After their year at a single site together, Megan, Maggie, Itzam, and Mallory exit the experimental clinical year and return to traditional clinical rotations, packing costume changes in the trunks of their cars for monthlong auditions in far-flung spots. They spend months at the university hospital across town but also at community hospitals across the state and at away rotations across the country. Some rotations are required, some are electives, and some are clinical auditions called acting internships, which amount to four weeks on an inpatient service acting as an intern, taking on the workload of an intern to prove their readiness. Ace the month, and you raise your odds of becoming a resident at that institution, in that specialty. Flub the audition, and doors close behind you. Exclusion and inclusion; kindergarten all over again.

After the relative safety of their clinical year together, the LIC students are traveling alone. They have individual work to do now, clinical rotations, but also applications to residencies, to secure their Match. They can apply in one specialty or several, to one program or dozens. If they earn an interview, they travel across the country, bedding in an alum's spare room or on a friend's sofa, then dressing up in an interview suit in a borrowed bathroom before enduring a daylong job interview, all to meet their Match.

While medical school graduation is a signal achievement, it makes you an MD, not a physician. Four years of your life is not enough to make you essential to the clinics and hospitals that need licensed and certified professionals. A medical school graduate needs to complete at least a one-year internship to earn an independent license. That makes you, at best, a general practitioner, which opens only a few doors. A physician needs to complete a residency of at least three years to become board eligible. Once board eligible, you can sit for another standardized exam, this one specific to the governing board of your specialty, whether it be niche like the American Board of Nuclear Medicine or something broader like the American Board of Family Medicine. (A physician can obtain multiple boards—Harvard's Dr. Hyun Joon Shin holds a world record for ten board certifications—if eligible.) Pass the board exam, and you are board certified. Many doors are opened for the licensed and certified.

The next door is the most important. Medical students seek their place in the internships and residencies that will make their careers through the Match. Mallory, Maggie, Megan, and Itzam will be 4 of the 40,084 applicants entering the year's Match and seeking entry into its 34,266 available internships [170, 171]. They are applying for programs that range from cutthroat competitive (e.g., neurosurgery, plastic surgery) to merely cut-wrist competitive (e.g., pediatrics, psychiatry). After a year of learning together in ungraded chalice exercises, the Match returns the LIC students to a world of meritocratic competition, of being evaluated on the merits of their work as isolated individuals.

The Match is the ultimate draft of meritocrats, even more so than something like the NBA draft, where basketball-playing adolescents from around the world are measured, interviewed, selected, and traded by plutocrats. The NBA draft is more egalitarian for programs—the worst teams have more opportunities to select the best prospects—and for applicants, who can delay their draft entry or play basketball in another league or sign as undrafted free agents.

This is not the case with the Match. Programs and applicants alike are contractually bound to use the Match as the only door to postgraduate training. The Match makes no attempt to redistribute the most promising future physicians to the communities that most need their services, instead concentrating the most promising physicians at the most established programs, even though graduate medical education is heavily subsidized by the federal government to serve community interests.

And, as befits meritocrats, the Match works on an economist's version of matchmaking, something called the Gale-Shapley algorithm. Before the algorithm's introduction, applicants and programs were often matched haphazardly. Some applicants were satisfied with the results, others were dissatisfied, and others were left unmatched. The economist Alvin Roth adapted the algorithm into the Match, transforming it into a sorting system that allows an applicant to find the program they most prefer from among the programs that prefer them [172, 173, 174].

Every applicant writes a rank list of programs—say, Dallas-Denver-Durham—usually including somewhere between five and twenty programs. Every program writes a rank list of applicants—say, Dwayne-Dolores-Declan. Applicants and programs certify their rank lists, and then the algorithm does the kind of matchmaking work that village elders once did. The algorithm attempts to place each applicant with their preferred program and each program with its preferred applicants. Sometimes a Dwayne settles for Dallas. Sometimes a Dolores gets Denver like she wanted. Sometimes a Declan goes unmatched.

Students do best when they rank more programs, when they score better on the Step 1 and 2 exams, and when they are inducted in the Alpha Omega Alpha Honor Medical Society—abbreviated AΩA and pronounced like a nonsense schoolyard chant *"ay-oh-ay"*—which affirms their place at the top of their medical school class. (Mackenzie and Mallory are both tapped for AΩA.) Attending an American medical school helps a great deal, and attending one of the country's leading research medical schools helps even more—a full third of the successful Matches are awarded to students at America's top forty research medical schools. Successful applicants report, on average, seven publications, three work experiences, three research experiences, and eight volunteer experiences [175]. But success falls along a spectrum. Only 46 percent of graduating American MDs will match to their first-choice program; 71 percent will match to one of their top three ranked programs. And even though the average applicant ranks thirteen programs, a full 6 percent of graduating MDs go unmatched [170].

It worked for Catherine Ard, the student in the year ahead. Catherine is staying in Colorado, at Denver Health, like she hoped. She will be able to follow the patients she met with Dr. Adams through residency. It was a Match with people as much as with the program. Now, the next class is seeking their own Match.

. . .

Students and faculty call it the Match, but Roth was always more plainspoken: it was a mathematical means of making a labor market more efficient [174], and his work eventually earned him the ultimate meritocrat's gold star: a Nobel Prize. It was in economics rather than medicine. The Match medical students pursue is, really, the market.

Two students opt out.

Sarah Bardwell goes south. She figures that leaving the clinic and the hospital is the best way to figure out her place in the strange worlds of medicine. At a minimum, she will learn Spanish. Her clinical year taught her that she needed the language to serve her future patients. "I really wanted to be able to provide medicine to Spanish-speaking patients in a way that I felt was equitable to them. I wish that everybody could have a doctor who spoke their language, but it's not possible in the United States." Sarah could make herself, at least, into that kind of physician.

Over six months she takes classes at the Universidad Nacional Autónoma de México and travels through Argentina and Chile, and then she spends six more weeks in Peru learning medical Spanish. She provides occasional health care, visiting places where an American fourth-year med student counts as a physician. She visits prisons and old folks' homes where English-speaking medical students from around the world set up shop and see thirty elderly people in an afternoon or fifty prisoners in a morning, the only care available.

"It's a shocking experience to walk into any kind of prison or jail. It's especially shocking in the women's prison; they have their kids in there with them. The kids don't spend all the time with them, but they get to spend like three to four days a week in the prison with their mom, especially little babies. So you have really, really rough conditions. People are being served food out of a 5-gallon plastic bucket that just sits on the ground. The bathrooms are filthy, toilets don't flush, there is no running water.

"Nobody in Peru has hot water in their house, so it changes the differential. There's no privacy, there's no way to do a thorough exam if someone has any kind of genital urinary symptoms, which was very common. People don't have fresh water to drink, so people are dehydrated. There's a lot of random overuse of antibiotics. A lot of women had chronic UTIs that were hard to treat. There's really no way to do any testing.

"You could do a urine sample for glucose, that's about it. There's no private place for people to do anything. There's no test so it's trying to figure out what people have, having a high suspicion of lots of terrible things, no ability to diagnose it, and then no way to refer them anywhere or do any tests. So essentially, we had a collection of fifty different medications that we could prescribe to people. And it's not, 'Oh, this person has high blood pressure. I'm going to give them a prescription for blood pressure medication.' It's, 'I can give them ten pills of a blood pressure medication.' And we won't have any more. The only way people get medications in these prisons is if someone from the outside brings it to them."

The experiences brought home to Sarah the privileges of American medicine, how even the privations of the patients at Denver

Health pale in comparison to what is available to the poor of Peru and Mexico.

"Being down there made me think, 'What are my goals?' Is it to serve the people who are most underserved? Because if so, I should be south of the border."

She planned to work in an urban environment, but the experience taught her that the need was greater in places remote from academic health centers. The homeless of Denver, she realized, had more access to advanced medicine than the people living in the rural communities she visited. It amplified her thoughts about the inequitable distribution of health care, about how the money of medicine gets in the way of the health of a community and how physicians become a part of that by giving up all their time for money. It sometimes seemed so beyond her ability to affect that it fueled a retreat to bourgeois thoughts— remodeling an old house, eating at tapas bars, buying a vacation house in the mountains.

"I feel serious shame that that is the kind of shit I think."

And she thought about how she would return to the States. She was no longer sure that she wanted to remain in Denver. The city had changed since her childhood, grown dense and expensive. Denver Health had changed too, from the scruffy hospital of her childhood into a place more polished. No longer sure where she fit in her hometown, Sarah would figure it out from afar.

. . .

Mackenzie Garcia also knew she wanted to leave her hometown, but with one more degree first, a master's of public health (MPH). She studied health care financing, policy, and systems management. She learned more about behavioral and community health, along with public health research methods. She found the health equity missing from medicine throughout her public health training.

"There is a larger medical culture of looking at biologic or genetic things causing health issues and not so much thinking about all of those social and structural issues around discrimination and historical and present-day injustices that lead to different health disparities."

When she began her MPH, Mackenzie had to shift her thinking from the patient level back to the societal level. Public health named structural barriers to health and strategized ways to break them down. Mackenzie loved the social-level analysis of public health. At the same time, she wanted to be a physician because it would allow her to relate to people on a more personal level.

Staying local for the degree allowed her to work regularly with one of her internal medicine preceptors—the same Dr. Sacro who gifted her with poetry—so she could maintain the relationship and her clinical skills. Mackenzie would be an internist too. She signed up for an acting internship, one of the monthlong clinical auditions a medical student undertakes in her final year, back at Denver Health. She loved the work of internal medicine, being a part of its team, but with the increased responsibility of a team member who had ascended to the next rung of the hierarchy. She even liked the chores of caring for patients on the medicine wards. Writing admission, progress, and discharge notes occupies most of the day for an acting intern. Mackenzie likes clinical tasks.

"It gives me a mechanism to be able to make sense of something in a world that doesn't necessarily always make that much sense. And it's kind of putting everything together and making sure that it addresses a whole patient and not just the one main reason they are in the hospital."

She liked the work enough that she considered staying home and training in the primary care internal medicine residency run by Dr. Sacro. After all, Catherine would be there, in the class ahead of

Mackenzie. The Denver Health program had almost everything she was looking for, almost a continuation of her student experiences, but she wondered about somewhere else.

...

The rest of the students were on track for the Match and enjoying the advertised version of the fourth year, at least at the start.

So was Dr. Adams. The months after one class finished was always the time for Kris Oatis to take a long vacation and for Adams to tinker with her curriculum before the next class arrived. This year, Adams was tinkering at scale. As her students were out auditioning, she was thinking about how she could teach the two textbooks to even more students. She started by flying Dr. David Hirsh out so he could introduce the LIC to all teachers at the medical school. She fills Hirsh's dance card: public lectures to build enthusiasm, departmental grand rounds to share evidence, and faculty workshops to strategize reform. In event after event, Hirsh asks the faculty what it would take for medical education to be a social good again. He shares that the LIC is a profoundly evidence-based and person-centered model, so it is a good way to provide a social good.

Since Hirsh first sketched out the LIC on a napkin with Dr. Ogur, he has found a variety of ways to explain the model, enlisting art, literature, philosophy, poetry, and science. It's a liberal arts version of medical education. The LIC's continuity with patients, peers, preceptors, and the public, Hirsh declares, allows students to remember medical knowledge in meaningful relationships [176]. Instead of the med students of old, whose rotating casts of preceptors peppered students with questions to assess their knowledge [177], Hirsh's LIC students fight the forgetting curve in relationships. They do it so well that Hirsh's model became essential to the future of medical training beyond Harvard [178], and Hirsh and Adams wonder whether it can be that way for Colorado as well.

In a small group of faculty members—Drs. Adams, Frank, and Kulasekaran are all in attendance—the angular and bespectacled Hirsh bounds about the room like a cut electric wire, sparked by being among his people, teaching physicians with Ogur's joy for the work. When faculty express skepticism about the LIC, he reassures them.

"I am not advocating the LIC itself but the LIC as a teaching model which enables medical education to be a social good. Education is a way to achieve what Aristotle calls the good, or human flourishing."

He offers a flurry of arguments about how education can respond to the ethical erosion observed among medical students in the clinical curriculum [179]. He speaks of an incongruity between the physicians we are training and what our community needs, and then he rattles off statistics. LIC students are more likely to see patients before and after they enter acute treatment. LIC students are more likely to report developing meaningful relationships with patients. LIC students are better prepared to enter today's workforce. LIC models can adapt to many systems and cultures. After getting statistical, Hirsh gets philosophical. He speaks about how the LIC fosters human flourishing, about how the teacher-student relationship can become a relationship of care analogous to the physician-patient relationship [180], about how students develop integrity because they participate in a relational learning model that aligns with their own core values and allows them to learn deeply [176], about how education can heal a fractured world, and about how the LIC induces conversation about what it means to educate someone well.

· · ·

The University of Colorado is all in. The university wants its students to flourish, to be engaged with their patients and their community. The medical school is considering a transformation of its entire curriculum, all four years, to teach the two textbooks. Hirsh celebrates the willingness to change the model for thousands of faculty and hundreds of students by embracing the LIC across the state.

"The LIC is exceptionally good at inducing conversation about what it means to educate someone. It is what the philosopher of science Thomas Kuhn calls a paradigm shift, a true step-up." Hirsh pauses to inhale a quick breath, then exhales it all as enthusiastic praise. "Schools often change their science or clinical curriculum. You are changing both simultaneously. It is frightening, but exciting. Your students are the luckiest people ever. This will make such a change for the students, the school, and your state."

Feeling it, he reads a *Lord of the Rings* quote to the gathered educators who will take on the many tasks of developing and implementing the new curriculum: "It is not our part to master all the tides of the world, but to do what is in us for the succor of those years wherein we are set, uprooting the evil in the fields that we know, so that those who live after may have clean earth to till. What weather they shall have is not ours to rule" [181, p. 160].

Now in full Gandalf mode, Hirsh delivers a noon-hour grand rounds, dispensing oracular wisdom to inspire the faculty for the journey ahead. They are, he fully believes, pursuing a better way to train tomorrow's physicians today if they follow the path Adams has pioneered at Denver Health.

. . .

Maggie is headed for med-peds and hopes to stay put at Denver Health. She knew that before her fourth year began, but getting there was momentous. Some med students do one acting internship; Maggie did three: medicine, medicine-pediatrics, and pediatrics itself. She loved each, even though she herself became a patient halfway through pediatrics.

"I got a pretty bad case of pneumonia and presented to the ER with four of four SIRS criteria, so I was hospitalized for a few days, getting IVs and antibiotics for that, which was eventful and exciting."

Maggie recovered but felt newly vulnerable to the respiratory diseases to which med-peds physicians are commonly exposed, and then she had to make up the week she missed later in the fall. Still, when the winter arrived, she was able to enjoy the fabled easiest year of school. She spent most of the winter skiing—she estimates fifty days on the slopes, more than earning her season pass—when she was not learning or traveling for interviews. She admits no angst. She is committed to med-peds.

What physicians in both disciplines share, Maggie believes, is a love for diagnostic puzzles, for doctoring as telling detective stories. Physicians in both specialties love not only being with their patients but also evaluating the available evidence. "When I think of people who work in both pediatrics and internal medicine, I think of people who are very warm and curious."

Just like the med-peds preceptor Dr. Anne Frank, toward whom Maggie felt so emulous.

So Maggie enters the Match as one of 606 applicants seeking one of the 390 positions in the nation's 77 med-peds programs [170, p. 10]. It is one of the most competitive specialties in the Match, but she enters the market intentionally, applying to only twelve of those programs after she vetted her list with her husband.

"It was a long conversation with him about where he would feel fulfilled and happy living. We looked at schools together."

Ten schools offered interviews; she accepted eight. Maggie went on interviews looking for the right fit. She loved them all, but home is what fits the homegrown Maggie. She knows that the training will change her, just like becoming a parent or a vampire, but she wants to change in place. To stay, she must stand out. The program accepts four interns, and there are four applicants from Colorado alone. The program is not allowed to tip its hand or ask her to tip her own. But she feels good about her prospects, about doctoring, and about her new name. Her married name is Kuusinen, a surname that means "son of spruce tree" in Finnish. A fitting name for somebody from the mountains like the soon-to-be Dr. Maggie Mae Kuusinen.

Despite her confidence, an announcement of her future is momentous enough to induce anxiety. Since her Match would affect them both, she plans to let her husband open her Match envelope.

"I am already such a ball of stress anyway that I just need his bravery to do that."

Transformative experiences require bravery because they ask you to give your life away to others, to radically recenter another person in your life through personal encounters. If becoming a physician is a transformative experience because being a physician means centering patients in your life, analogous to hearing what you previously could not hear, to parenting a child who arrives as a stranger, or to committing to caring for a spouse in sickness and health, then all of medicine was about to be transformed. So before Maggie could borrow her husband's bravery, before Megan could sit at a table with her family, the whole world became a ball of stress, as the COVID-19 epidemic erupted.

Chapter 26

ESSENTIAL WORKERS

THE STUDENTS MUST DECIDE if they will become vampires or heroes.

While her classmates were flying around the country for acting internships and residency interviews, Sarah Bardwell was out of the country, distancing herself from medical training. Too much about medical school felt like a constant climb up a hierarchy that distanced a physician from her patients. She wondered how to collapse the distance between patient and physician. When the pandemic arrived, Sarah felt like it overwhelmed that defensive fantasy, revealing that people were vulnerable in ways that had been repressed. The defensive fantasy was part of why Sarah needed a year away from American medicine to find her future within it.

As Sarah traveled to clarify her goals, the SARS-CoV-2 virus was advancing along flight paths, and people began asking her questions about the virus.

"People were really scared. So I spent a lot of time talking with people about my perspective, which was wrong 50 percent of the time because I'd never seen a pandemic before."

Sarah could acknowledge her inexperience, the limits of a fourth-year student's knowledge. But she was shocked by the responses of people she thought would know better.

"I thought that world governments had their shit more together. I think a lot of people have been really shocked to see the utter mismanagement, the complete lack of intelligent thinking that has happened."

She planned another month in Guatemala, but Guatemala began closing its borders, and Sarah checked the United States Embassy website daily, concluding that it was time to head home. She took two cabs and two buses to Mexico City International Airport. Usually one of the world's busiest, it was empty this time. When her plane touched down in Denver, everything seemed changed.

Epidemiologists had counseled quarantine. The city was shuttered. It frightened her, but Sarah felt a little like she had the city of her childhood back. The traffic abated, so the smog had cleared. She breathed better and saw the mountains more clearly than in decades. The pandemic had emptied Denver's streets.

The pandemic filled the hospitals. The treatments were supportive: fluids, oxygen, ventilators. Speculators proposed timeworn treatments—artemisia, betel, cannabis, chloroform, datura, fennel, methanol, turmeric—and profited from them. Physicians admitted patients who drank bleach as a speculative treatment, only to discover that it burned out their esophagus, not the virus.

. . .

Epidemiologists kept on trying to fit the outbreaks caused by SARS-CoV-2 into clear models, but the virus seemed haphazard, irregular, and random. When SARS-CoV-2 became the COVID-19 pandemic, epidemiologists counseled social distancing, and it seemed like an egalitarian treatment. *Everyone should keep six feet apart. Everyone should mask. Everyone should stay home if sick. Everyone should work together.* But it quickly became clear that social distancing was not available for those already at society's margins. It was easier to stay six feet apart, mask, stay home, and work together if you owned your own dwelling and could work online. The professional class—attorneys, engineers, financiers—could often work remotely. The essential workers—first responders, grocers, nurses, postal workers—could not work from home. The institutionalized—prisoners, homeless—could neither work nor be at home.

Physicians cared for the institutionalized while straddling the professional-essential divide.

For all of medicine's current decadence, physicians were essential workers, like custodians, because much of the work had to be done in person. In a rare moment, the lives of meritocrats met the working class. Physicians left their children home alone and went every day to the hospital before dawn, which quickly became even more somber than usual. Visitors were restricted. Beds were filled. Toilet paper was stolen from staff bathrooms. Personal protective equipment became as a rare as a moment of peace. Physicians texted each other pictures of themselves swathed in whatever armor they could assemble against an invisible virus. Sometimes it was a full kit of protective booties, face shield, gloves, gown, and mask. Often, it was only a cloth mask.

When they left the hospital, they listened to the communal wolf calls that carried out over the city, whose trees bore signs of support for essential workers. They watched as fireworks celebrated masked heroes. It felt, in Maggie's phrase, that the world needed to borrow bravery.

Denver Health felt more like the field hospital it once was. Physicians drew up plans for turning a bare parking lot—catering tents over patient beds lined up in parking spaces previously reserved for commuters' cars—into a makeshift hospital. Leadership entered incident command, a hierarchical structure that focused everyone's efforts against the pandemic. Physician leaders spoke of waging trench warfare against the virus by putting boots on the ground, reinforcing the martial metaphors undergirding medicine. *Doctor's orders, operating theaters, surgical fields.* Dutiful combatants raised hands to work with the infected, while conscientious objectors sought alternative service. It was hero time.

Society agreed. Around town, the plywood sheets covering closed restaurants became canvases for murals of masked clinicians, arms crossed over green scrubs, hands sheathed in sparring gloves, angel wings sprouting from their scapulae. Giant heart stickers, with the word "HOPE" in the middle, were wheat-pasted to neighborhood garages and to the walls of the hospital wards. Quarantined community members sewed homemade masks, dropping off boxloads of stitched protective gear for the workers at the front. Shuttered restaurants cooked down the food in their refrigerators, delivering baked goods and coffee to clinical workrooms just behind the front lines. In each bite and sip, physicians could taste the nearness between health care workers and the community, the solidarity between a community and its health care workers.

Each act of solidarity fueled health care workers who problem-solved treatments as the patient beds filled. Physicians learned to use heated and high-flow oxygen for the infected and, while awaiting the vaccine, scoured the available pharmaceutical armamentarium, finding success with dexamethasone and remdesivir. Health care workers spent months with the ill, as they lingered on ventilators, their families forbidden to visit. When patients recovered enough for discharge, the hospital would play a celebratory pop song over the hospital intercom, but then the copyright holder threatened a lawsuit, so the hospital settled on a chime. When patients succumbed, the hospital silently added names to the unfurling list of victims. Life had a sound; death was silent.

Early in the pandemic, there was a feeling of being fully a physician, as every action was about caring for the most ill and preventing the spread of illness in a community, instead of generating vulgar profits for health care factories. Despite the very real dangers of doctoring in that moment, physicians felt, however briefly, like the kind of elegant and fabulous vampires Paul describes. Physicians lived with unbridled enthusiasm. Some mistook it for heroism.

. . .

Not Sarah. She worried about what the pandemic would bear. She saw friends lose their businesses. She feared that they would never recover. She saw the pandemic accelerating changes.

"It's going to be devastating for a long time. I think it's really pushed forward a lot of the changes in labor that we've been on the cusp of in the United States. I fear what it's done to our hospital systems and what we're going to see, the fallout of the pandemic is going to. I can't even conceptualize that yet, but I know that it's there."

Sarah knew it would take more than a one-time rescue operation to save medicine. As she progressed in her medical training, she saw that so much was wrong. The pandemic made health care jobs simultaneously less secure and more demanding. Further levels of disenchantment seemed likely. There was talk of a vaccine built on mRNA technology, a startlingly effective advance straight from the textbook-of-the-body approach to medicine, but it was already being politicized in ways that revealed how much distrust and polarization were sickening our communities.

And yet, Sarah was too far along to quit her dream. Somehow, during the pandemic, Sarah would complete her fourth year, interview for a family medicine residency position, and chart her entry into a changing, charged world.

. . .

While Sarah comes home, Mackenzie Garcia must stay home.

The medical school and the hospital issue pandemic declarations, filling out just four blank lines on a single-page form, checking one box, and sending it off to the accrediting body for medical education. Upon its receipt, the accrediting body acknowledges that the usual version of medical education—clinical rotations, classroom lectures, and faculty evaluations—must change. The pandemic shutters the clinics and operating rooms where clinical education occurred, so long-deferred

changes arrive for medical education. Resident physicians are rede-
ployed to the front lines, hospital wards and intensive care units that
care for the infected, instead of to their usual clinical assignments. Unlike a century ago, when most medical students were conscripted into
clinical work to function autonomously as physicians, only a few medical schools graduate students early so they can doctor on the pandemic's front lines [182, 183]. Most medical students are dismissed from
clinical rotations. Step 1—the exam that stratifies students—becomes a
pass/fail exam. Medical student admission interviews and resident
recruiting trips both become virtual.

With clinical rotations canceled and examinations altered, some
students take the opportunity to become something beyond learners.
They organize community donations, manage volunteers, sew masks,
march in the streets. Others, like Mackenzie, become part of a group of
medical students who are, suddenly, essential. Although she works
from home to avoid exposing loved ones to the virus, she uses her
clinical skills and public health knowledge to inform the hospital's
leadership. When the hospital begins daily briefings, med students
are not only in the room where the decisions are made; they run the
presentations. Med students are the ones who have the time to gather
and synthesize information. Med students are the ones who share the
competing epidemiological models predicting the pandemic's projected
peaks and troughs. Meanwhile, the interns in the year ahead of them,
like Catherine Ard, work clinically on the COVID wards.

Mackenzie finds that having essential work helps manage the increased anxieties that accompany the pandemic: "It gives me something tangible to do: contributing to a larger picture." As soon as she
starts hearing about the novel virus, Mackenzie joins a group of medical
students who volunteer to help. She starts checking daily case counts
from the state's public health department and sharing the information
in an online newsletter for the public. She reads medical journals from

the United States and China and synthesizes the information, translating medicalese into patient language like Dr. Stichman taught her. Mackenzie brings forward both her clinical and public health training to fight the pandemic, even as she awaits her own fate.

. . .

When physicians like Dr. Ard left the hospital each night, they would take off their N95 masks to reveal visible rashes, in the shielding shape of a mask. Raised pandemic pimples felt like the erupting signs of a more vital medical practice. They felt encouraged when someone graffitied "H-E-R-O-E-S" on the side of a hospital building. Entering each morning, they smiled ruefully at the suggestion that it applied to them.

What do heroes do?

Save the day.

This worked for the first few months, when experts thought that the pandemic would follow the projected curve of a tragedy, from disaster to reconstruction, within a year. But as reconstruction was delayed and delayed again, when supplies were eventually restored but staff grew shorter and shorter, physicians realized they didn't need heroes to save the day, because the day was adding up to weeks and months and years. They didn't need heroes for that work.

They needed the kind of vampires Paul spoke of.

Dr. Ard was becoming one because, like many physicians in training, she was reassigned to intensive care units where patients lingered for months on ventilators, their families forbidden to visit, only to die a medicalized death. Other physicians reviewed the records of every patient who died with COVID in those months. When they added up the cases—*a grandmother with diabetes, a grandson with an amputated leg, an uncle with hypertension, a cousin with leukemia*—it sounded like a roll call. The virus's randomness resolved. In some neighborhoods, people worked from home. In other neighborhoods, people were livestreaming funerals.

COVID-19 was not haphazard or random, but precisely sickening and killing the people who lived at the margins of the city. Cases concentrated in neighborhoods north and west of Denver's Inverted L. Deaths were concentrated in the city's minority populations, especially its Latino community [184]. The city and the hospital gradually moved from alliance (*We are all in this together!*) to anxiety (*Who will survive this?*) to anger (*Why are some surviving this differently?*) to anguish (*Why are some losing so much?*). The weaknesses in every system—agricultural, biological, economic, environmental, legislative, political—were exploited by merely one of the thirty-nine known species of coronaviruses. The United States had invested in high-tech medicine, but it was low-tech measures—social distancing, handwashing, universal masking, essential workers—that society needed. The vulnerabilities of the community allowed a microscopic virus to humble a superpower, with the tragic result that while the United States contained 4 percent of the world's population, it experienced 20 percent of its COVID fatalities [185].

Every preexisting condition, every social determinant of health added up together to determine who was affected, who got sick, who lost work, who lost housing, and who died. Barely a month into the shutdown, it became clear that COVID was as precise a market as the Match: the virus exploited every inequality across a community, including a medicine built up from the textbook of the body.

. . .

The LIC graduation meal, in a crowded break room of a hospital, was supposed to be a foretaste of the students' Match Day ballroom banquet. Instead, their dress rehearsal from the year before became the last ceremony they shared in person. COVID canceled communal meals like banquets. Instead of an in-person ballroom, the students meet up for a livestream of a gathering of medical school deans seated in a suburban dining room. The faculty are waiting for the Match to release the fates of the students waiting in their own dwellings.

To help the students pass the fifteen minutes until the students, along with every medical student across the country, learn their fate, the deans tell their own Match stories.

An internist talks about how he couples-matched from halfway across the country. He tied his own entry in the Gale-Shapley algorithm with a classmate, a strategy often undertaken by a married couple, but which can be undertaken by anyone who desires to shorten their odds and raise their stakes to include both personal and professional satisfaction. The Match sorted them from Dartmouth to Colorado and made his career.

Dr. Zimmer interviewed at internal medicine programs all over the country before settling on a suicide match (med school lingo for entering a single choice into the Match). Her physician fiancé was at Emory, so she ranked Emory and Emory alone. She tells the students that she was at brunch, drinking mimosas, a few days before Match Day when she began to worry. "My mother had told me, 'Be a leader, not a follower,' and in that moment, I realized that for the first time in my life I had followed someone else." She acknowledged that many students chose where to Match based not just on their own needs but on the needs of their family.

An emergency medicine physician talks about his disappointing Match Day. His suicide match failed, leaving him scrambling for a spot in a busy one-year surgical training program in Hawaii. He never learned to surf, but he learned that the Match you didn't want could sometimes be better than the one you sought.

Another internist says that, like this year's med students, she also missed her Match Day. She was on an away rotation. She ranked only two programs and received her first choice but celebrated it as a visiting med student in an unfamiliar hospital, before returning to work.

The deans reassure the students watching at home. "We could tell you countless stories about folks who did not get the Match they desired and eventually concluded it was the best thing that ever happened."

Disappointment could, they promise, be transmuted into gratitude. The students waiting for their fates are praying they will never have to learn those lessons. With their fiancé or spouse or sister at their side, Itzam, Maggie, Mallory, and Megan are anxious to know where they will train.

The deans finally give the signal, the envelopes open, and the students begin texting their news to the deans, announcing the full range of teaching hospitals: *Saint Joseph, Sinai, Stanford.*

Amid the callouts, Maggie texts in. "I love you all so much. Thank you so much for the support through the years. Congratulations!" She was staying in Colorado. Medicine-pediatrics. She voted on her relationships. They voted back: yes. It was a Match to cry tears of joy over.

Megan cries too. "So proud of this incredible class for everyone's support and resilience," she texts. She will be known as a physician. After sending out speculum valentines to the world, it sent back a career as an obstetrician. She is headed to Creighton, away from her boyfriend, for OB-GYN.

Itzam is not traveling after all. A father now, he goes full Disney for the group text: "*Hakuna matata* to everyone." Itzam, Andrea, and their infant, Itziara, stay in Colorado for ophthalmology.

Mallory completes the Couples Match. She and her fiancé match at the same hospital, affiliated with Baylor, her undergraduate alma mater. A different kind of homecoming. Her fiancé will be a general surgeon, and she, an internist. She is even thinking, in a final triumph over her childhood fear of blood, of becoming a hematologist-oncologist.

Within a half hour, the livestream is over, a land speed record for a Match Day celebration.

This year, the real celebrations occur when the screens are closed. Most of the students stay in their rented apartments and family homes, wherever they received their fate, even in backyards and emptied city parks, where more than a few of the mimosas Zimmer mentioned are sipped. Not the LIC students. They head for the public health building's LIC classroom, where they shared so many chalice exercises, to be together again. Itzam, Maggie, Mallory, and Megan link arms with other LIC students, lean into the camera, and smile their relief at meeting their Match, so their picture can join the framed alumni portraits on the grandmother wall.

But first, Dr. Adams sends the pictures out to her LIC alumni and faculty to announce their Match. "Today our fifth cohort of LIC students matched into residencies so I want to share their great news with you!" Adams spent the day with her matching students, celebrating their past and processing their futures. She dreams that some might return as faculty.

Work interrupts her dreams. She will be at the hospital all weekend, rearranging the present for the next class. The pandemic is worsening, canceling all formal med student rotations, and she is patching together a plan, so that the next group of students can find the same satisfaction on their own Match Day. She has more futures to realize, more physicians to train for tomorrow. She cannot wait until tomorrow. She starts again the same day.

. . .

So does Kris Oatis. She collects badges from med students who are soon to graduate and returns them to security. One of them reads "Mallory Myers, Medical Student." Since Mallory will be a physician soon, she needs a physician's badge instead. More access, more status, more demands. Mallory proved she could do the work, so she would have more work. Oatis, a definite people person, misses the students and is dealing with her own pandemic disappointments. She cancels a trip for which she spent years saving money and vacation days. But she is soldiering on, helping the students who come after Mallory make their own progress through the strange worlds of medicine.

The faculty members were still teaching, but mostly virtually. After decades of lecturing in large auditoriums with banked seats extending two stories up, trying to reach the whole room by asking questions and greeting students, the faculty are teaching online. Instead of looking into 184 faces, they gaze into 184 tiny blanked screens across a Zoom screen. For some faculty, the experience leaves them wondering why they teach. The physician's quotidian opening question—*What brings you here?*—is a medical question and an existential question. Giving a lecture during a pandemic surfaces the existential questions, but teaching online leaves you alone with those questions. There are no students hanging about afterward to ask more questions, helping to clarify a thought or qualify a comment over a cup of coffee.

Teaching while socially distanced feels impersonal to the point of alienation. Some faculty realize that this was what the people they met as patients had been trying to tell them for years before the pandemic: we are all too distant from each other.

Like Sarah suspected, the pandemic accelerates change. Within the med school, the push to transform the curriculum gains momentum. The old curriculum seems even more outmoded in a pandemic of infection and inequality. Dr. Adams gets the call for which she has been waiting.

Adams has so expertly shown the success of the LIC at Denver Health that the medical school has endorsed the LIC as its future. Adams is amassing data comparing her dozens of LIC students to more than a thousand students in the school's regular training program. The LIC students are more likely to serve their community, while just as likely to know how to care for the bodies of their patients. More than 70 percent of her LIC students were working in urban underserved settings like Denver Health, and nearly all of them remained committed to working in medically underserved communities [186]. Teaching the two textbooks works so well that the senior associate dean of education, Dr. Zimmer, has decided that all Colorado medical students will be trained in an LIC.

Over the next three years, Zimmer will lead a change from a curriculum that Osler and Flexner would have recognized—two years of basic sciences, a clinical year of rotating clerkships, and a final year of specialization—to one comprising four years of integrated work. The new curriculum will begin with a year of basic sciences but will be organized around clinical complaints. Hence, instead of learning the anatomy of the heart as its own topic, students will learn it in the context of a patient presenting with chest pain [187]. They will learn about the anatomy of the heart in relationship to the physical examination, to available medications and procedures, and to social determinants of health. They will learn the textbook of the body, Zimmer hopes, while learning the textbook of the community. She will have to recruit and train 1,100 faculty members so that all students' second year can be an LIC year. Students will be split into sixteen cohorts spread across the state. Three of the cohorts will occur at Denver Health; Drs. Adams, Frank, and Kulasekaran will each lead one of these cohorts. The new curriculum's third year will be an advanced science year, in which students will begin specializing: a future neonatologist might study more genetics; a future neurologist might study more neurosciences. The new curriculum's fourth year will be a capstone year, with advanced clinical and science rotations as preparation for their chosen specialty.

In the Flexnerian era, medical students were treated like passive recipients, empty vessels to be filled with scientific knowledge. Zimmer welcomes today's students as active partners who shape the curriculum. The medical school adopts a series of virtues—leadership, curiosity, commitment—to guide their medical students as they develop a physician's practical wisdom. Zimmer envisions the curriculum as a conversation with students, faculty, and the community, not something delivered from above, and she has recruited a legion of colleagues and collaborators.

The model will allow Adams and Zimmer to extend the LIC's vision across all four years. Students will engage in the care of some of their patients over their entire clinical years, with the same preceptors, in a continuous relationship. Students will achieve their clinical competencies across multiple disciplines simultaneously. Students will receive their lessons at the kind of intervals Ebbinghaus found best reinforced learning.

All the faculty must do is redesign all the curricular material and retrain a couple thousand faculty members to teach differently. During a pandemic. Since Zimmer placed Adams in charge of the clinical curriculum that will alter the lives of every academic physician and medical student in the state, Adams will organize it. Instead of intimately supervising the clinical education of a couple handfuls of students, in a year's time she will direct the clinical education of 736 students.

. . .

By staying for residency, Catherine was advancing Adams's dream of creating another generation of physicians for their community. Staying allowed Catherine to follow Cecilia, a patient they shared, through med school and into residency. Now, Catherine is already planning to stay for her first faculty job. As Adams moves into the dean's office, Catherine might even take over Adams's place as a primary care physician at one of the clinics. "It's humbling," Catherine says. "I think she was one of the best primary care doctors. All of her patients love her. It really challenges me to be a better doctor." Catherine thought about what made Adams the doctor she wanted to emulate.

"She has a way of sitting down with her patients and kind of connecting with them in just a couple of minutes. She sits down and really makes them feel like they're seen and heard. She's a very strong advocate for her patients."

When Catherine sees a patient on her own, she finds that "I have this 'What would Jen Adams do?' voice in the back of my head." The voice often tells her to do more, to advocate more, for the patient. "She really advocates for her patients, so that they can get the best care that they can get. I want to bring more of that to my practice. I hope to be the type of doctor that Jen Adams kind of taught me to be. I hope to maybe see if I can bring any more changes to Denver Health. I love Denver Health but I think there are some ways that we can kind of expand and grow and become more involved with the community."

Adams has formed Catherine into someone committed to knowing, ever better, how to serve the bodies and communities of her patients. Now Catherine wants to teach herself, to extend the bridge that Adams offered. Now Catherine is becoming her own bridge to the future of medicine.

Catherine, like the majority of her LIC students, will fulfill Adams's dream of training physicians and educators for a different kind of medicine. Adams knows that Catherine, Itzam, Mackenzie, Mallory, Megan, and Sarah are putting themselves forward as physicians. The students proved themselves ready by bettering other people's lives because teachers like Adams first bettered the students' lives. The LIC created a relationship where the faculty saw the students, so the students could the see the patients. The faculty gave lessons, counsel, balls of yarn, even poetry.

There is another poem, "Little Owl," by A. E. Stallings, which begins, "It's not what we see, but what sees us / Makes us who we are" [188]. The moments when the students were seen occurred when they truly met other people and bettered their lives. Those moments bettered the students' own lives in return. They flourished, together, when they were able to build relationships over time. L-I-C still, after all, rhymes with "Now, I see."

ESPERANZA

$\mathcal{G}$RADUATION DAY ARRIVES. The campus quad is usually filled with proud parents, their soon-to-be physician children, and faculty dressed in medieval-era doctoral gowns, trimmed in green for medicine. Dr. Adams would usually be decked out, but is instead driving around Denver, delivering gloves, gowns, and masks to area hospitals. The limited supply of personal protective equipment is the rate-limiting step for allowing medical students to learn at the hospitals. She wants students on the front lines, so she delivers the equipment herself.

The Zoom ceremony starts without her. The chancellor accepts the list of graduates from the deans of each health profession school. The university's president offers congratulatory words. The students break out into a separate ceremony just for medical students. Most of the deans from Match Day speak at the graduation, but this time the students speak too.

The class president speaks about how their education was disrupted. He teases classmates who have grown COVID beards or given themselves home haircuts. He calls out classmates who, watching graduation from their couches, are wearing pajamas underneath their robes and keeping a mimosa (or two) just out of the camera's view.

His jokes land, but the graduation speech genre requires earnest reflection, so the class president also speaks about how medical students showed grit throughout their training but sacrificed even more during the pandemic. On their screens, the students look somber. The students realize that they became essential. They were called heroes, even though they really needed to be more like vampires. Now they will become physicians.

After the class president, a few more deans speak, and then the dean of the university himself, a pulmonologist and critical care physician who knows what a pandemic respiratory illness can do to patients and society alike, takes the stage and welcomes the graduates to the ranks of physicians.

"In 1972, two famous paleontologists, Niles Eldredge and Stephen Jay Gould, published a very influential paper on evolution, entitled 'Punctuated Equilibrium.' And in that paper, they postulated that rather than a continuous gradual change, evolution was characterized by abrupt changes, followed by a period of relative stability. And I would put to you that this COVID pandemic is one of those abrupt changes."

The dean asks the students to prepare themselves for living in a moment of terrific change, of punctuated equilibrium. Medical education and practice will change, and it will change quickly now. The event, stripped of its usual ceremony, proceeds just as quickly. The graduates are announced, via title slides, trimmed in the school's black and gold colors, which give their name, their future, and a brief message from the graduate.

Megan Elizabeth Kalata, MD. "I am exceedingly grateful to my family and incredible mentors for your guidance, patience, and unwavering support during this journey. Thank you!"

Maggie Mae Kuusinen, MD. "Sean—I could not have done this without you. I love you. Grandma Barb—I am here because of you. Family, friends, mentors—thank you for everything."

Alejandro Itzam Marin, MD. "This, I owe it to my wife and best friend Andrea. You and Itziara, you give me strength. Thanks for the immeasurable support of my family and friends."

Mallory Elizabeth Myers, MD. "Thank you to my parents, husband, mentors, and friends for your unconditional love and support. I couldn't have done it without you!"

And with that message, Mallory lets a secret slip. Adams texts her. *Husband?* Mallory admits that when the pandemic delayed her wedding, she and her fiancé-classmate eloped. They were together in the Match, and now they are together in marriage. That ceremony will wait—and wait again and again, thrice delayed by the pandemic—but the marriage is already realized.

The only remaining thing to do is to swear on it.

Dr. Zimmer takes the virtual stage. "This promise, as a physician's oath, is something that you should savor. Our physician father, Hippocrates, unifies us in the practice of medicine, the most amazing calling and privilege."

As Zimmer invokes Hippocrates, I am alone in my office, thinking of Sarah Bardwell and Mackenzie Garcia, still a year away from their own graduation. (Sarah will alight for rural Idaho, to train as a family physician in a setting more like the Denver of her childhood than the Denver of today. Mackenzie will move to Atlanta, to train in internal medicine at Emory, one of the leading medical schools for bridging public health and clinical medicine.) I think of Catherine Ard, already fighting the pandemic in her first year of internship. (At the end of the pandemic, she will indeed take over Adams's former clinical role, fulfilling Adams's dream of making doctors for her patients, and Dr. Ard will start her own journey as an attending physician.) I think of the new students coming behind them. I think of all the physicians I know. I think of all the physicians laboring away in intensive care units while I watch graduation. I think of all my friends sickened by the virus. I think of the hundreds of health care workers who died caring for patients. I think of the hundreds of thousands of patients who are dying.

I reach for a collection of aphorisms attributed to Hippocrates, gifted to me at my own medical school graduation. I read again this counsel: "For the medical man sees terrible sights, touches unpleasant things, and the misfortunes of others bring a harvest of sorrows that are peculiarly his; but the sick by means of the art rid themselves of the worst of evils, disease, suffering, pain and death" [189, p. 227].

Did these newest physicians know what they were swearing to? Did any of us?

I began thinking of all that will need to change as the pandemic ends. We will have to do it together. We will have to rebuild social trust across the divisions exposed and exacerbated by the pandemic. We will have to serve those with the greatest need in their local community. We will have to do it in the small rooms where people can meet each other across divisions. We will have to do it in a way that valorizes talents beyond the ability to climb up our inequity-increasing meritocracy [190, 191].

In the end, Hirsh is right: the LIC is simply one way to do that within medical education, a way to teach two textbooks. Every hospital that hosts an LIC will have their own curricular focus; their own Dr. Jen Adamses and Kris Oatises will bless each program with its own flavor. Their students will, like Itzam, Maggie, Mackenzie, Mallory, Megan, and Sarah, have the chance to prove themselves together, within a longitudinal curriculum built on relationships—around personal encounters between students and patients, students and faculty—that uses time as a tool.

Encounters over time become the kind of relationships that build you into a different person, a person capable of being a physician to someone else, a person who knows the body and the community, and a person whose actions advance the health of both. A person who deserves to be known as a physician.

As they become physicians, students often worry that they are, themselves, impostors. They doubt themselves. They fear that people will find out that they are incapable of the work. It is common among med students [192]. It is also common among their faculty [193]. After all, they are both locked into an educational system that can feel like a performance [194]. The doctor's life can feel like one performance after another, pretending through it all.

In the end, all of us pretend to be physicians. To be human is to pretend. We put ourselves forward in social roles. Patient, then student. Student, then physician. Physician, then patient again. Each comes with different names to represent those identities. Eventually, if you pretend long enough, it becomes a social identity that displaces your first name: Doctor.

Dr. Kalata. Dr. Kuusinen. Dr. Marin. Dr. Myers. Dr. Bardwell. Dr. Garcia.

The name symbolizes a new way of putting yourself forward in the world.

But when we put ourselves forward as physicians, we know that our pretending may fall short of what the name proposes us to be.

I know, down deep, that in putting myself forward as a physician, I fall short of being a physician, a person qualified to heal. Who can truly heal another person's body or a community?

I also know that medicine is a life in which the distance between schadenfreude and success can be vanishing.

As you become a physician, you learn to delight in the ways a body falters and fails. You come to admire the extremes of pathology. You swap stories of impolitic speech and heroic overdoses and sprawling tumors. But then you have to somehow remember that the patient before you is a person like your forgivable brother, your irresistible ex-ex, your endearingly shaggy neighbor. To succeed, you must acknowledge that sometimes you feel like an impostor and sometimes like a professional, sometimes inadequate to that day's performance and sometimes closer to being a person truly worthy of caring for another person.

We need a social structure that brings physicians a little closer to being worthy. We need a system where students follow patients instead of professionals. We need a system that makes physicians better instead of beating them up. We need a possible way through a collapsing culture. We need a system where visiting a patient in their home is more important than dissecting a corpse. We need medical students to learn the social determinants of health along with the derangements of pathophysiology. We need to build wise practitioners instead of meritocrats and technocrats. We need more primary care physicians instead of subspecialist physicians. We need a system that measures skills instead of exam scores. We need a system that truly includes people from all backgrounds, so we have the natural attorneys for those with the greatest needs. We need a system that everyone can afford, so that it enriches physicians and patients alike. We need a system that prioritizes both justice and efficiency. We need a system that trains physicians to work downstream, where disease presents, and upstream, at the social causes of disease. We need a system that enchants again and allows physicians to truly flourish, to realize their potential by caring well for patients.

A global pandemic that exploited health inequalities, social divisions, and disenchanted professionals drove home the lesson that individuals are well only when the community is well, that we need clinical medicine and public health, in a version of medicine that truly asks what is in "the general interest of the community." The LIC is a step toward building a health care system that serves a community's general interest. Students follow patients instead of physicians. Students build relationships over time with those patients and with a committed group of faculty members. Students learn through team-based chalice exercises instead of individual cram sessions. Students rotate between specialties every day instead of every few months so that they can integrate medical knowledge across the artificial lines between specialties. It's a curriculum built on continuity and relationships. It's two textbooks instead of one. But it's still a textbook approach, instead of a full collaboration with a community, a true accompaniment between physicians and the people they meet as patients. Perhaps it's the step we can take now in medical education, knowing that the next step toward full collaboration is the one that will truly make us the physician a community needs.

The LIC step may be difficult enough. It requires dedicated teachers and administrators, the Kris and Jen team in every hospital, to coordinate all the steps. It requires new curricular materials. It requires reeducation of the faculty. It is a difficult change.

Training physicians is difficult for all these reasons, but even more, it is difficult because being a human is difficult. We make progress only in hindsight. We see who we have become only at the story's end. To be alive, you must put yourself forward in some fashion. Putting yourself forward as a physician means you put yourself forward while putting your patients forward as well. A good physician flourishes only when their patients flourish and when their students are sent forward into the future to continue the work of doctoring.

Zimmer invites the students to stand, unmute themselves, and read a version of the oath together.

Unmuting and switching their videos on, the graduates reveal their celebration scenes. Some sit on gaming couches. Some hold cozied beers or whiskey tumblers. Some stand before virtual backdrops of the beaches to which they cannot travel during quarantine. Some hold children, some stand alone in their living rooms, and some sit with their parents. For once, they are all unmasked. As the students see each other, they mock each other's hair and shoes and outfits.

I glimpse Dr. Kuusinen standing—where else?—outside, gowned in long black robes trimmed with green. Dr. Kalata is standing—where else?—with her sister, arm in arm, to swear their oaths together.

Zimmer invites the faculty watching to recite along with the students. Without thinking, I stand and recite with them.

> I swear by what is sacred to me that I will fulfill, according
> to my ability and judgment, this oath and this covenant:
> I devote myself to the health of humanity, with full respect
> for the dignity and worth of each person. Above all, I will
> strive to do no harm.
> I recognize that my knowledge and skills are imperfect,
> and that I must always seek further training and growth.
> I will not perform treatments for which I am not qualified,
> and I will call upon others for help. In turn, I will gladly
> render aid when asked.
> I commit myself to the profession of medicine, to the
> advancement of scientific knowledge, and to the education
> and mentorship of those who follow me.
> I will respect the rights of my patients and colleagues and
> shall safeguard those confidences placed in me.
> I will speak out when silence is wrong. I will respect the law,
> but I will not fail to seek changes that would reduce suffering
> or contribute to good health.
> I recognize the trust that has been placed in me by society
> and by my colleagues. I will at all times comport myself
> with dignity, honesty, humility, and integrity.
> These things I do swear solemnly, freely, and upon my
> personal and professional honor.

As we finish, Zimmer says, "Many things have been canceled in the last few months. *La esperanza no ha sido cancelada.* Hope has not been canceled."

Zimmer looks directly at her screen so she can address the graduates—students no more—as physicians. "Welcome to the profession of medicine. Your patients have been waiting for you."

Alone in my office, I close the computer and cry. My first real pandemic tears. Undignified, unceremonious. Through those tears, I could see all that we were doing. I see that, even during a pandemic, the students proved themselves.

I write Zimmer an email and thank her. She writes back immediately.

"What a day. Indeed. Thank you for joining them! I always feel that ceremonies bind us together and it almost felt more meaningful to do it knowing we were all over the country and in our separate spaces across the School. Together."

Still crying, I call my wife.

She spent the previous night, sleepless, on call. We speak of our own graduation. It was in person, on a sunny day. Our parents attended. Our infant son perched in our arms. Three generations. The day felt like a goodbye to our student days and a hello to a future promising good work with each other and with the ill and with our community. Fifteen years later, watching the newest future physicians and joining their oath taking from a distance, it still does.

Acknowledgments

A week after completing residency, I joined Denver Health because Dr. Bob House promised me I would see underserved patients, teach the next generation of physicians how to care for them better than I do, and write about my experiences. He was right. I am grateful daily for the opportunities the patients, staff, and faculty at Denver Health afford me. As I wrote this book, the following Denver Health people were especially helpful: Kathy Beauchamp, Dennis Boyle, Kathy Boyle, Lynne Briggs, Peg Burnette, Vince Collins, Chawtana Edwards, Danielle Foley, Patricia Gabow, Jama Goers, Tereza Guedes, Mike Haley, Simon Hambidge, LaToya Hammons, Mario Harding, Romana Hasnia-Wynia, Jonathan Hawkins, Robert House, Bonnie Kaplan, Amanda Klahr, Donna Lynne, Tom Mackenzie, Sarah Meadows, Maria Moreira, Liana Patterson, Connie Price, Laura Rendon, Maria Schimpf, Scott Simpson, La Vaughn Standridge, Natalia Villalba, Melissa Weiser-Rose, Helena Winston, and Chelsea Wolf.

At the University of Colorado School of Medicine, Eva Aagaard, Brenda Bucklin, Austin Butterfield, John Reilly, Carol Rumack, Joe Sakai, Darlene Tad-y, Nichole Zehnder, and Shanta Zimmer inspired me with their passion and rigor for medical education. Tara Bannon Williamson and all the staff at the Park Hill branch of the Denver Public Library provided stacks of books and archival material. The members of our local writing group—Matt

Allen, Rob Broadhurst, Nathaniel Brown, Peter Coleman, Steven Huett, Mark Kissler, and Josh Williams—kept me afloat with rotator beers, canny counsel, and sustaining friendship. Bridget Rector and Elin Kondrad read and improved the first draft. Mia Alvarado and Melissa Musick tolerated my interim drafts. Jon Cox and Susan Ginsburg bettered the second draft, helping me translate the strange world of medicine.

At Johns Hopkins University Press, Robin Coleman realized the promise of the resulting book. His encouraging words and formative criticism transformed the manuscript.

Other friends, in Denver and abroad, who encouraged this book include Andrew Ciferni, Farr Curlin, Lydia Dugdale, Jeff Haanen, Robert Hilt, Warren Kinghorn, Brett McCarty, T. R. Reid, Helen Thorpe, and Sophia Wang.

I deeply thank Catherine Ard, Sarah Bardwell, Mackenzie Garcia, Megan Kalata, Maggie Kuusinen (née Kriz), Itzam Marin, and Mallory Smith (née Myers), who allowed me to use their names and quote our encounters. Each of these students reviewed and improved the text before publication. Their teachers, especially Jennifer Adams, Jennie Buchanan, Kurt Cook, John (Jack) Cunningham, Stefka Fabbri, Anne Frank, Phil Fung, Kshama Jaiswal, Vishnu Kulasekaran, Anna-Lisa Munson, Kristina Oatis, Yasmin Sacro, Jennifer Stichman, and Meg Tomcho, are my betters. Watching a fellow physician work is a kind of professional intimacy, seeing how a peer cares for patients and teaches their students. From each of these preceptors, I learned to be a better physician.

No one encouraged the writing of this book more than Elin Kondrad. It's a matter of dispute when we first met, but we have been talking to each other every day since the first day of medical school. She can tell you stories of practicing sutures on beggared beef from the butcher, of holding necrotic limbs while fighting back morning sickness, and of being stuck with infected needles while pregnant. She survived a serious car crash, a complicated delivery, and marriage to me, all while becoming a remarkable family medicine physician and residency program director. Her work is the story behind this story. Twenty years in, there is still no one else with whom I would rather travel the strange worlds of medicine and marriage, and no one to whom I am more grateful.

We hold our place in the world as physicians only for a time. Our work is to make it better and hand it off. Since the future of medicine remains contested and worth fighting for, a portion of the proceeds of this book support the Sabin Scholarship at Denver Health.

References

1. Association of American Medical Colleges, *2021 fall applicant, matriculant, and enrollment data tables*. 2021, Washington, DC: Association of American Medical Colleges.

2. Ginzberg, E., and H.S. Berliner, *Teaching hospitals and the urban poor*. 2000, New Haven, CT: Yale University Press.

3. King, M., *A spirit of charity: Restoring the bond between America and its public hospitals*. 2016, Salisbury, MD: Secant.

4. Hafferty, F.W., *Into the valley: Death and the socialization of medical students*. 1991, New Haven, CT: Yale University Press.

5. Dugdale, D.C., R. Epstein, and S.Z. Pantilat, *Time and the patient-physician relationship*. J Gen Intern Med, 1999. 14(Suppl. 1): S34-40.

6. Horace, *The complete Odes and Epodes: With the Centennial hymn*. Penguin classics. 1983, New York: Penguin.

7. *Health Services Integration*. 1982, Washington, DC: National Academies Press.

8. Welsome, E., *A dream delivered: The community health center movement in Denver from the Civil Rights Act to the Affordable Care Act*. 2016, Denver: Denver Community Health Services.

9. Richards, E., *The Knife and Gun Club: Scenes from an emergency room*. 1989, New York: Atlantic Monthly Press.

10. Kraft, L., *Ned Wynkoop and the lonely road from Sand Creek*. 2011, Norman: University of Oklahoma Press.

11. Welsome, E., *Healers and hellraisers: Denver Health's first 150 years*. 2011, Denver: Denver Health Foundation.

12. Swenson, P.A., *Disorder: A history of reform, reaction, and money in American medicine*. 2021, New Haven, CT: Yale University Press.

13. Barr, D.A., *Questioning the premedical paradigm: Enhancing diversity in the medical profession a century after the Flexner Report*. 2010, Baltimore: Johns Hopkins University Press.

14. Flexner, A., Carnegie Foundation for the Advancement of Teaching, and H.S. Pritchett, *Medical education in the United States and Canada; a report to the Carnegie Foundation for the Advancement of Teaching*. 1910, New York: Carnegie Foundation for the Advancement of Teaching.

15. Morantz-Sanchez, R.M., *Sympathy and science: Women physicians in American medicine*. 1985, New York: Oxford University Press.

16. Gatchel, J., et al., *Neurosyphilis in psychiatric practice: A case-based discussion of clinical evaluation and diagnosis*. Gen Hosp Psychiatry, 2015. 37(5): 459–63.

17. Swain, K., *"Extraordinarily arduous and fraught with danger": Syphilis, Salvarsan, and general paresis of the insane*. Lancet Psychiatry, 2018. 5(9): 702–3.

18. Rothstein, W.G., *American medical schools and the practice of medicine: A history*. 1987, New York: Oxford University Press.

19. Walsh, M.R., *"Doctors wanted, no women need apply": Sexual barriers in the medical profession, 1835–1975*. 1977, New Haven, CT: Yale University Press.

20. Ludmerer, K.M., *Let me heal: The opportunity to preserve excellence in American medicine*. 2015, New York: Oxford University Press.

21. Morsy, L., *Carnegie and Rockefeller's philanthropic legacy: Exclusion of African Americans from medicine*. Acad Med, 2023. 98(3): 313–16.

22. Dante, A., R. Pinsky, and N. Pinsky, *The Inferno of Dante: A new verse translation*. 1994, New York: Farrar, Straus & Giroux.

23. Boethius and D.C. Langston, *The consolation of philosophy: Authoritative text, contexts, criticism*. 1st ed. Norton critical editions in the history of ideas. 2010, New York: W. W. Norton.

24. Montgomery, K., *How doctors think: Clinical judgment and the practice of medicine*. 2006, Oxford: Oxford University Press.

25. US Preventive Services Task Force, *A and B Recommendations*. 2020. https://www.uspreventiveservicestaskforce.org/uspstf /recommendation-topics/uspstf-a-and-b-recommendations.

26. US Preventive Services Task Force et al., *Screening for prostate cancer: US Preventive Services Task Force recommendation statement*. JAMA, 2018. 319(18): 1901-13.

27. Kapoor, D.A., *A history of the United States Preventive Services Task Force: Its expanding authority and need for reform*. J Urol, 2018. 199(1): 37-39.

28. Aronowitz, R., and J.A. Greene, *Contingent knowledge and looping effects—a 66-year-old man with PSA-detected prostate cancer and regrets*. N Engl J Med, 2019. 381(12): 1093-96.

29. Levy, B.S., and V.W. Sidel, *Social injustice and public health*. 2006, Oxford: Oxford University Press.

30. Sandomir, R., *Dr. Victor Sidel, public health champion, is dead at 86*. *New York Times*, February 7, 2018.

31. Remington, P.L., B.B. Catlin, and K.P. Gennuso, *The County Health Rankings: Rationale and methods*. Popul Health Metr, 2015. 13(1): 11.

32. Sobel, R.K., *MSL—medicine as a second language*. N Engl J Med, 2005. 352(19): 1945-46.

33. Kalter, L., *U.S. medical school enrollment rises 30%*. 2019, Washington, DC: Association of American Medical Colleges.

34. IHS Markit Ltd., *The complexities of physician supply and demand: Projections from 2018 to 2033*. 2020, Washington, DC: Association of American Medical Colleges.

35. Osler, W., *A way of life*. 1925, London: Constable.

36. Osler, W., *Aequanimitas*. 2nd ed. 1914, Philadelphia: P. Blakinson's Son.

37. Bryan, C.S., *The influence of Sir Andrew Clark (1826-93) on William Osler (1849-1919)*. J Med Biogr, 2005. 13(4): 195-200.

38. US Food and Drug Administration, *FDA at a glance*. 2020, Silver Spring, MD: US Food and Drug Administration.

39. Hüllen, W., *A history of Roget's Thesaurus: Origins, development, and design*. 2004, Oxford: Oxford University Press.

40. Dewey, J., *Experience and education*. 1938, New York: Macmillan.

41. Hirsh, D.A., et al., *"Continuity" as an organizing principle for clinical education reform*. N Engl J Med, 2007. 356(8): 858-66.

42. Ogur, B., et al., *The Harvard Medical School-Cambridge integrated clerkship: An innovative model of clinical education*. Acad Med, 2007. 82(4): 397-404.

43. Strasser, R., and D. Hirsh, *Longitudinal integrated clerkships: Transforming medical education worldwide?* Med Educ, 2011. 45(5): 436-37.

44. Hirsh, D., et al., *Educational outcomes of the Harvard Medical School-Cambridge integrated clerkship: A way forward for medical education*. Acad Med, 2012. 87(5): 643-50.

45. Walters, L., et al., *Outcomes of longitudinal integrated clinical placements for students, clinicians and society*. Med Educ, 2012. 46(11): 1028-41.

46. Gaufberg, E., et al., *Into the future: Patient-centredness endures in longitudinal integrated clerkship graduates*. Med Educ, 2014. 48(6): 572-82.

47. Norris, T.E., et al., *Longitudinal integrated clerkships for medical students: An innovation adopted by medical schools in Australia,*

Canada, South Africa, and the United States. Acad Med, 2009. 84(7): 902–7.

48. Barzansky, B.M., N. Gevitz, and College of Medicine at Chicago, *Beyond Flexner: Medical education in the twentieth century.* 1992, New York: Greenwood.

49. Miller, B.M., et al., *Beyond Flexner: A new model for continuous learning in the health professions.* Acad Med, 2010. 85(2): 266–72.

50. Cooke, M., et al., *Educating physicians: A call for reform of medical school and residency.* 1st ed. 2010, San Francisco: Jossey-Bass.

51. World Health Assembly, *Edinburgh declaration on the reform of medical education.* 1989, Geneva: World Health Organization.

52. Bloom, S.W., *The medical school as a social organization: The sources of resistance to change.* Med Educ, 1989. 23(3): 228–41.

53. Gheihman, G., et al., *A review of longitudinal clinical programs in US medical schools.* Med Educ Online, 2018. 23(1): 1444900.

54. Mazotti, L., et al., *Diffusion of innovation and longitudinal integrated clerkships: Results of the clerkship directors in internal medicine annual survey.* Med Teach, 2019. 41(3): 347–53.

55. Burnett, K.E., et al., *Longitudinal integrated foundation training: Uplifting perspectives.* Med Educ, 2018. 52(11): 1205.

56. Poncelet, A.N., et al., *Creating a longitudinal integrated clerkship with mutual benefits for an academic medical center and a community health system.* Perm J, 2014. 18(2): 50–56.

57. Poncelet, A., et al., *Development of a longitudinal integrated clerkship at an academic medical center.* Med Educ Online, 2011. 16: 10.3402/meo.v16i0.5939.

58. Worley, P., et al., *A typology of longitudinal integrated clerkships.* Med Educ, 2016. 50(9): 922–32.

59. Hirsh, D., L. Walters, and A.N. Poncelet, *Better learning, better doctors, better delivery system: Possibilities from a case study of longitudinal integrated clerkships.* Med Teach, 2012. 34(7): 548–54.

60. Hirsh, D., and P. Worley, *Better learning, better doctors, better community: How transforming clinical education can help repair society.* Med Educ, 2013. 47(9): 942–49.

61. Tennyson, A.T., and N. Page, *Alfred Lord Tennyson: Selected poetry.* 1995, London: Routledge.

62. Beck, J.S., *Cognitive therapy: Basics and beyond.* 1995, New York: Guilford.

63. Shanafelt, T.D., et al., *Burnout and satisfaction with work-life balance among US physicians relative to the general US population.* Arch Intern Med, 2012. 172(18): 1377–85.

64. Shanafelt, T.D., et al., *Changes in burnout and satisfaction with work-life balance in physicians and the general US working population between 2011 and 2014.* Mayo Clin Proc, 2015. 90(12): 1600–1613.

65. Gold, K.J., A. Sen, and T.L. Schwenk, *Details on suicide among US physicians: Data from the National Violent Death Reporting System.* Gen Hosp Psychiatry, 2013. 35(1): 45–49.

66. Eisenstein, L., *To fight burnout, organize.* N Engl J Med, 2018. 379(6): 509–11.

67. Elton, C., *Also human: The inner lives of doctors.* 1st ed. 2018, New York: Basic Books.

68. Prentice, S., et al., *Burnout levels and patterns in postgraduate medical trainees: A systematic review and meta-analysis.* Acad Med, 2020. 95(9): 1444–54.

69. Winston, H., and B. Fage, *Resilience, resistance: A commentary on the historical origins of resilience and wellness initiatives.* Psychiatr Serv, 2019. 70(8): 737–39.

70. Hojat, M., et al., *The devil is in the third year: A longitudinal study of erosion of empathy in medical school.* Acad Med, 2009. 84(9): 1182–91.

71. Newton, B.W., et al., *Is there hardening of the heart during medical school?* Acad Med, 2008. 83(3): 244–49.

72. Dyrbye, L.N., M.R. Thomas, and T.D. Shanafelt, *Systematic review of depression, anxiety, and other indicators of psychological distress among U.S. and Canadian medical students.* Acad Med, 2006. 81(4): 354–73.

73. Dyrbye, L.N., et al., *Relationship between burnout and professional conduct and attitudes among US medical students.* JAMA, 2010. 304(11): 1173–80.

74. Dyrbye, L.N., et al., *Burnout and suicidal ideation among U.S. medical students.* Ann Intern Med, 2008. 149(5): 334–41.

75. Nussbaum, A.M., *I work in a locked psych ward. These days, you do too.* Stat, 2021. https://www.statnews.com/2021/12/23/i-work-in-a-locked -psychiatric-ward-these-days-you-do-too/.

76. Adams, J., et al., *Reflective writing as a window on medical students' professional identity development in a longitudinal integrated clerkship.* Teach Learn Med, 2020. 32(2): 117–25.

77. Wellbery, C., et al., *Medical students' empathy for vulnerable groups: Results from a survey and reflective writing assignment.* Acad Med, 2017. 92(12): 1709–14.

78. Flick, R.J., et al., *Alliance, trust, and loss: Experiences of patients cared for by students in a longitudinal integrated clerkship.* Acad Med, 2019. 94(11): 1806–13.

79. Brown, M.E.L., et al., *Medical student identity construction within longitudinal integrated clerkships: An international, longitudinal qualitative study.* Acad Med, 2022. 97(9): 1385–92.

80. Sacks, O., *Hallucinations.* 1st American ed. 2012, New York: Alfred A. Knopf.

81. Sinsky, C., et al., *Allocation of physician time in ambulatory practice: A time and motion study in 4 specialties.* Ann Intern Med, 2016. 165(11): 753–60.

82. Association of American Medical Colleges, *Tuition and student fees report, 2012-2013 through 2019-2020.* 2021, Washington, DC: Association of American Medical Colleges.

83. Papanicolas, I., L.R. Woskie, and A.K. Jha, *Health care spending in the United States and other high-income countries.* JAMA, 2018. 319(10): 1024–39.

84. Anderson, G.F., P. Hussey, and V. Petrosyan, *It's still the prices, stupid: Why the US spends so much on health care, and a tribute to Uwe Reinhardt.* Health Aff (Millwood), 2019. 38(1): 87–95.

85. Shrank, W.H., T.L. Rogstad, and N. Parekh, *Waste in the US health care system: Estimated costs and potential for savings.* JAMA, 2019. 322(15): 1501–9.

86. Ludmerer, K.M., *Time to heal: American medical education from the turn of the century to the era of managed care.* 1999, New York: Oxford University Press.

87. Association of American Medical Colleges, *AAMC faculty salary survey.* 2019, Washington, DC: Association of American Medical Colleges.

88. National Education Association, *Estimates of school statistics, selected years, 1969–70 through 2016–17,* in *Digest of Education Statistics.* 2017, Washington, DC: National Center for Education Statistics, Institute of Education Sciences, U.S. Department of Education. https://nces.ed.gov/pubs2018/2018070.pdf.

89. Steinbrook, R., *Easing the shortage in adult primary care—is it all about money?* N Engl J Med, 2009. 360(26): 2696–99.

90. Rohlfing, J., et al., *Medical student debt and major life choices other than specialty.* Med Educ Online, 2014. 19: 25603.

91. Youngclaus, J., S.A. Bunton, and J. Fresne, *An updated look at attendance cost and medical student debt at U.S. medical schools,* in *Analysis in Brief.* 2017, Washington, DC: Association of American Medical Colleges. https://www.aamc.org/data-reports/analysis -brief/report/updated-look-attendance-cost-and-medical-student -debt-us-medical-schools.

92. Grischkan, J., et al., *Distribution of medical education debt by specialty, 2010–2016.* JAMA Intern Med, 2017. 177(10): 1532–35.

93. Youngclaus, J., and L. Roskovensky, *An updated look at the economic diversity of U.S. medical students*, in *Analysis in Brief*. 2018, Washington, DC: Association of American Medical Colleges.

94. Zhang, D., et al., *Trends in medical school application and matriculation rates across the United States from 2001 to 2015: Implications for health disparities*. Acad Med, 2021. 96(6): 885–93.

95. Piketty, T. *Brahmin left vs merchant right: Rising inequality and the changing structure of political conflict*. 2018. PSE Working Papers hal-02878211, HAL.

96. Lautenberger, D.M., and V.M. Dandar, *The state of women in academic medicine 2018-2019: Exploring pathways to equity*. 2020, Washington, DC: Association of American Medical Colleges.

97. Boyle, P. *What's your specialty? New data show the choices of America's doctors by gender, race, and age*. 2023, Washington, DC: Association of American Medical Colleges.

98. Anonymous, *Florence Rena Sabin, "first lady" of Colorado*. JAMA, 1963. 186: 1090–91.

99. Bluemel, E., *Florence Sabin: Colorado woman of the century*. 1959, Boulder: University of Colorado Press.

100. Rosof, P.J.F., *The quiet feminism of Dr. Florence Sabin: Helping women achieve in science and medicine*. Gender Forum, 2009. 2009(24): 33–55.

101. Sabin, F.R., and H.M. Knower, *An atlas of the medulla and midbrain*. 1901, Baltimore: Friedenwald.

102. Sabin, F.R., *The origin and development of the lymphatic system*. 1913, Baltimore: Johns Hopkins Press.

103. Sabin, F.R., *The people win for public health in Colorado*. Am J Public Health Nations Health, 1947. 37(10): 1311–16.

104. Hunter, R.C., J.G. Lohrenz, and A.E. Schwartzman, *Nosophobia and hypochondriasis in medical students*. J Nerv Ment Dis, 1964. 139: 147–52.

105. Adrian, C., *The children's hospital*. 2006, San Francisco: McSweeney's Books.

106. Webster, R.K., et al., *A systematic review of infectious illness presenteeism: Prevalence, reasons and risk factors*. BMC Public Health, 2019. 19(1): 799.

107. Szymczak, J.E., et al., *Reasons why physicians and advanced practice clinicians work while sick: A mixed-methods analysis*. JAMA Pediatr, 2015. 169(9): 815-21.

108. Rosvold, E.O., and E. Bjertness, *Physicians who do not take sick leave: Hazardous heroes?* Scand J Public Health, 2001. 29(1): 71-75.

109. Klitzman, R., *When doctors become patients*. 2008, Oxford: Oxford University Press.

110. McKenna, T.J., *Graves' disease*. Lancet, 2001. 357(9270): 1793-96.

111. Anonymous, *Longevity of persons engaged in different occupations*. Scientific American, 1858. 13(47): 371.

112. Frank, E., H. Biola, and C.A. Burnett, *Mortality rates and causes among U.S. physicians*. Am J Prev Med, 2000. 19(3): 155-59.

113. Duarte, D., et al., *Male and female physician suicidality: A systematic review and meta-analysis*. JAMA Psychiatry, 2020. 77(6): 587-97.

114. Setiya, K., *Midlife: A philosophical guide*. 2017, Princeton, NJ: Princeton University Press.

115. Goldacre, M.J., J.M. Davidson, and T.W. Lambert, *Doctors' age at domestic partnership and parenthood: Cohort studies*. J R Soc Med, 2012. 105(9): 390-99.

116. Shanafelt, T.D., et al., *The medical marriage: A national survey of the spouses/partners of US physicians*. Mayo Clin Proc, 2013. 88(3): 216-25.

117. Ly, D.P., S.A. Seabury, and A.B. Jena, *Divorce among physicians and other healthcare professionals in the United States: Analysis of census survey data*. BMJ, 2015. 350: h706.

118. Isaac, C., et al., *Male spouses of women physicians: Communication, compromise, and carving out time*. Qual Rep, 2013. 18: 1-12.

119. Schrager, S., A. Kolan, and S.L. Dottl, *Is that your pager or mine: A survey of women academic family physicians in dual physician families.* WMJ, 2007. 106(5): 251-55.

120. Stentz, N.C., et al., *Fertility and childbearing among American female physicians.* J Womens Health (Larchmt), 2016. 25(10): 1059-65.

121. Lawrence-Lightfoot, S., *Balm in Gilead: Journey of a healer.* Radcliffe biography series. 1988, Reading, MA: Addison-Wesley.

122. Teherani, A., et al., *Burden, responsibility, and reward: Preceptor experiences with the continuity of teaching in a longitudinal integrated clerkship.* Acad Med, 2009. 84(Suppl. 10): S50-53.

123. Snow, S.C., J. Gong, and J.E. Adams, *Faculty experience and engagement in a longitudinal integrated clerkship.* Med Teach, 2017. 39(5): 527-34.

124. Shakeri, A., *Filippo Pacini—a life of achievement.* JAMA Dermatol, 2018. 154(3): 300.

125. Fitzharris, L., *The butchering art.* 1st ed. 2017, New York: Scientific American / Farrar, Straus & Giroux.

126. Best, C.H., *Diabetes and insulin and the lipotropic factors.* American lecture series. 1948, Springfield, IL: C. C. Thomas.

127. Eisenberg, D.S., *How hard it is seeing what is in front of your eyes.* Cell, 2018. 174(1): 8-11.

128. James, W., and M.H.P.T. Machado, *Brazil through the eyes of William James: Letters, diaries, and drawings, 1865-1866.* Bilingual ed. 2006, Cambridge, MA: Harvard University, David Rockefeller Center for Latin American Studies.

129. Guevara, C., and A. Wright, *The motorcycle diaries: A journey around South America.* 1995, London: Verso.

130. Du Mez, K.K., *A new gospel for women: Katharine Bushnell and the challenge of Christian feminism.* 2015, Oxford: Oxford University Press.

131. Perekrestov, E., *Alexander Schmorell: Saint of the German resistance.* 2017, Jordanville, NY: Holy Trinity, Printshop of St Job of Pochaev.

132. Kidder, T., *Mountains beyond mountains*. 1st ed. 2003, New York: Random House.

133. Bannister, R., *The four minute mile*. 1955, New York: Dodd, Mead.

134. Bannister, R., *Twin tracks: The autobiography*. 2014, London: Robson.

135. Murre, J.M., and J. Dros, *Replication and analysis of Ebbinghaus' forgetting curve*. PLoS One, 2015. 10(7): e0120644.

136. Association of American Medical Colleges, *Medical school graduation questionnaire 2020: All schools summary report*. 2020, Washington, DC: Association of American Medical Colleges.

137. Oser, T.K., et al., *Frequency and negative impact of medical student mistreatment based on specialty choice: A longitudinal study*. Acad Med, 2014. 89(5): 755–61.

138. Marin, M., et al., *Measles transmission and vaccine effectiveness during a large outbreak on a densely populated island: Implications for vaccination policy*. Clin Infect Dis, 2006. 42(3): 315–19.

139. Neyman, J., and H. Jeffreys, *Outline of a theory of statistical estimation based on the classical theory of probability*. Philos Trans Royal Soc A, 1997. 236(767): 333–80.

140. Sandercock, P.A., *Short history of confidence intervals: Or, don't ask "Does the treatment work?" but "How sure are you that it works?"* Stroke, 2015. 46(8): e184–87.

141. Weber, M., and J.E.T. Eldridge, *Max Weber: The interpretation of social reality*. Tutor books. 1970, London: Joseph.

142. Nussbaum, A.M., *The worthless remains of a physician's calling: Max Weber, William Osler, and the last virtue of physicians*. Theor Med Bioeth, 2018. 39(6): 419–29.

143. Weber, M., et al., *The vocation lectures*. 2004, Indianapolis: Hackett.

144. Madison, D.L., *Review of "Osler: Inspirations from a great physician," by Charles S. Bryan*. N Engl J Med, 1997. 337(18): 1324–26.

145. Bean, W.B., *The student life*. Arch Intern Med, 1959. 103(1): 168–69.

146. Anderson, G.A., *Charity: The place of the poor in the biblical tradition*. 2013, New Haven, CT: Yale University Press.

147. Risse, G.B., *Mending bodies, saving souls: A history of hospitals*. 1999, New York: Oxford University Press.

148. Case, A., and A. Deaton, *Deaths of despair and the future of capitalism*. 2020, Princeton, NJ: Princeton University Press.

149. Anonymous, *Pioneer woman doctor struggles and reaches top: Colorado's first doctor of color passes after 50 years of service. Denver Star*, October 18, 1952.

150. Anadiotis, K.A., *Justina Ford: Baby doctor*. Great lives in Colorado history. 2013, Palmer Lake, CO: Filter.

151. Harris, M., *The forty years of Justina Ford. Negro Digest*, March 1950, 42–45.

152. Farmer, P., and J. Weigel, *To repair the world: Paul Farmer speaks to the next generation*. 2013, Berkeley: University of California Press.

153. Farmer, P., *Pathologies of power: Health, human rights, and the new war on the poor*. California series in public anthropology. 2003, Berkeley: University of California Press.

154. Obermeyer, Z., et al., *Dissecting racial bias in an algorithm used to manage the health of populations*. Science, 2019. 366(6464): 447–53.

155. Vyas, D.A., L.G. Eisenstein, and D.S. Jones, *Hidden in plain sight—reconsidering the use of race correction in clinical algorithms*. N Engl J Med, 2020. 383(9): 874–82.

156. Williams, D.R., J.A. Lawrence, and B.A. Davis, *Racism and health: Evidence and needed research*. Annu Rev Public Health, 2019. 40: 105–25.

157. Tollette, W.Y., *Justina Lorena Ford, M.D.: Colorado's first black woman doctor*. 2005, Denver: Western Images.

158. Baker, R.B., et al., *Creating a segregated medical profession: African American physicians and organized medicine, 1846–1910*. J Natl Med Assoc, 2009. 101(6): 501–12.

159. Harley, E.H., *The forgotten history of defunct black medical schools in the 19th and 20th centuries and the impact of the Flexner Report.* J Natl Med Assoc, 2006. 98(9): 1425–29.

160. Wilson, D.E., *Minorities and the medical profession: A historical perspective and analysis of current and future trends.* J Natl Med Assoc, 1986. 78(3): 177–80.

161. Johnson, L.W., Jr., *History of the education of Negro physicians.* J Med Educ, 1967. 42(5): 439–46.

162. Association of American Medical Colleges, *Diversity in medicine: Facts and figures 2019.* 2019, Washington, DC: Association of American Medical Colleges.

163. Lohse, J.B., *Justina Ford, medical pioneer.* A now you know bio. 2004, Palmer Lake, CO: Filter.

164. Epps, C.H., Jr., D.G. Johnson, and A.L. Vaughan, *Black medical pioneers: African-American "firsts" in academic and organized medicine. Part one.* J Natl Med Assoc, 1993. 85(8): 629–44.

165. Association of American Medical Colleges, *Resident report.* 2019, Washington, DC: Association of American Medical Colleges.

166. Aciman, A., *Call me by your name.* 1st ed. 2007, New York: Farrar, Straus & Giroux.

167. Kaur, R., *Milk and honey.* 2015, Kansas City, MO: Andrews McMeel.

168. Paul, L.A., *Transformative experience.* 1st ed. 2014, Oxford: Oxford University Press.

169. Morrissette, A., and M. Morrissette, *"The feeling of failure is immense": A qualitative analysis of the experiences of unmatched residency applicants using Reddit.* Acad Med, 2023. 98(5): 623–28.

170. National Resident Matching Program, *Results and data: 2020 main residency Match®.* 2020, Washington, DC: National Resident Matching Program.

171. National Resident Matching Program, *Charting outcomes in the Match: Senior students of U.S. medical schools, 2020.* 2020, Washington, DC: National Resident Matching Program.

172. Roth, A.E., *New physicians: A natural experiment in market organization.* Science, 1990. 250(4987): 1524-28.

173. Roth, A.E., and E. Peranson, *The effects of the change in the NRMP matching algorithm. National Resident Matching Program.* JAMA, 1997. 278(9): 729-32.

174. Roth, A.E., *The economics of matching: Stability and incentive.* Math Oper Res, 1982. 7(4): 617-28.

175. National Resident Matching Program, *Charting outcomes in the Match: Senior students of U.S. medical schools, 2020.* 2020, Washington, DC: National Resident Matching Program.

176. Gaufberg, E., et al., *In pursuit of educational integrity: Professional identity formation in the Harvard Medical School Cambridge Integrated Clerkship.* Perspect Biol Med, 2017. 60(2): 258-74.

177. Nagarur, A., et al., *Words matter: Removing the word pimp from medical education discourse.* Am J Med, 2019. 132(12): e813-14.

178. Schwartzstein, R.M., et al., *The Harvard Medical School Pathways curriculum: Reimagining developmentally appropriate medical education for contemporary learners.* Acad Med, 2020. 95(11): 1687-95.

179. Hafferty, F.W., and J.F. O'Donnell, *The hidden curriculum in health professional education.* 2014, Hanover, NH: Dartmouth College Press.

180. Balmer, D.F., et al., *Caring to care: Applying Noddings' philosophy to medical education.* Acad Med, 2016. 91(12): 1618-21.

181. Tolkien, J.R.R., *The return of the king: Being the third part of the lord of the rings.* 2001, Boston: Houghton Mifflin.

182. Harrison, N.J., A.J. Schaffer, and D.W. Brady, *Comparing and contrasting the experiences of U.S. medical students during the COVID-19 and 1918 influenza pandemics.* Acad Med, 2023. 98(5): 555-62.

183. Goldberg, E., *Life on the line: Young doctors come of age in a pandemic.* 2021, New York: Harper.

184. Podewils, L.J., et al., *Disproportionate incidence of COVID-19 infection, hospitalizations, and deaths among persons identifying as Hispanic or Latino—Denver, Colorado March-October 2020.* MMWR Morb Mortal Wkly Rep, 2020. 69(48): 1812–16.

185. Wright, L., *The plague year: America in the time of COVID.* 2021, New York: Alfred A. Knopf.

186. Adams, J.E., et al., *Preliminary workforce outcomes of an urban longitudinal integrated clerkship.* Acad Med, 2023. 98(12): 1420–27.

187. Mandin, H., et al., *Developing a "clinical presentation" curriculum at the University of Calgary.* Acad Med, 1995. 70(3): 186–93.

188. Stallings, A.E., *Like: Poems.* 2015, New York: Farrar, Straus & Giroux.

189. Hippocrates and W.H.S. Jones, *Hippocrates.* The Loeb Classical Library. 1923, London: Heinemann.

190. Appiah, A., *The lies that bind: Rethinking identity, creed, country, color, class, culture.* 2018, New York: Liveright.

191. Sandel, M.J., *The tyranny of merit: What's become of the common good?* 2020, New York: Farrar, Straus & Giroux.

192. Villwock, J.A., et al., *Impostor syndrome and burnout among American medical students: A pilot study.* Int J Med Educ, 2016. 7: 364–69.

193. LaDonna, K.A., S. Ginsburg, and C. Watling, *"Rising to the level of your incompetence": What physicians' self-assessment of their performance reveals about the imposter syndrome in medicine.* Acad Med, 2018. 93(5): 763–68.

194. Tompkins, J.P., *Pedagogy of the distressed.* College English, 1990. 52: 121–30.

Index

acting internships, 242, 323, 326

Adams, Jennifer: Ard on, 342–43; author's experience with, 8–9; background, 111–13; and community service project, 96–97; and complex systems, 91; and COVID-19, 339, 344; and diversity of students, 296; and feet checks, 240, 249; on harm, 217; health of, 25, 205, 207; and HIV patients, 115, 301; LIC development, 9–10, 35–36; LIC expansion, 234–35, 324–26, 340–42; LIC faculty recruitment, 226; LIC graduation, 302, 305–10; LIC orientation, 36, 37–47, 141–43; LIC student recruitment, 116; marriage, 218; and Match announcement, 339; medical training, 113–15, 183; on mental health of students, 141–43; and patient-physician relationship, 18–22, 27–31, 119–20; as preceptor, 240, 309; and self-disciplining strategies, 279; social determinants focus, 57–58;

speed of seeing patients, 110; teamwork with Oatis, 122, 123, 124–25, 136; time pressures as primary care physician, 18–31

addiction medicine, 153

advanced practice providers, 263–64

Aequanimitas (Osler), 277

Alpha Omega Alpha Honor Medical Society, 319

altered mental status lesson, 255–57

altruism, 280–82, 284, 307–8

American Medical Association Council on Medical Education, 51

anal wink, 205

anesthesiology, 102, 182

antibiotics, 54

apprenticeship model of medical education, 50, 120

Ard, Catherine: on Adams, 342–43; background, 95–97, 155–56, 160–61; community service project, 94–97, 289; and COVID-19, 334, 335, 346; as LIC instructor/mentor, 38, 94–97;

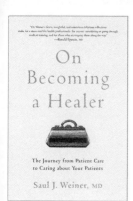

"From a wise doctor dedicated to a life of service, a vital and practical guide on how to be human in medicine. It goes to the core of our mission—to nourish the rising of a mutual relationship as the essence of healing."

—**Samuel Shem, MD,**
author of *The House of God*

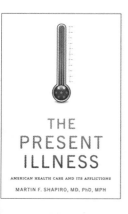

"Powerfully and originally explores the politics and economics of American health care. Required reading for anyone who seeks to know more about how we got sick and wants to imagine how on earth we can begin to get better."

—**Jonathan Metzl,**
author of *Dying of Whiteness*

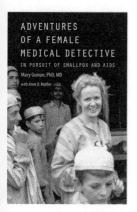

"A rip-roaring read. As a 'medical detective,' Guinan presents a series of case studies in explicit homage to super-sleuth Sherlock Holmes."

—*Nature*

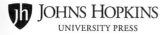